THE BOOK OF CHAKRA HEALING

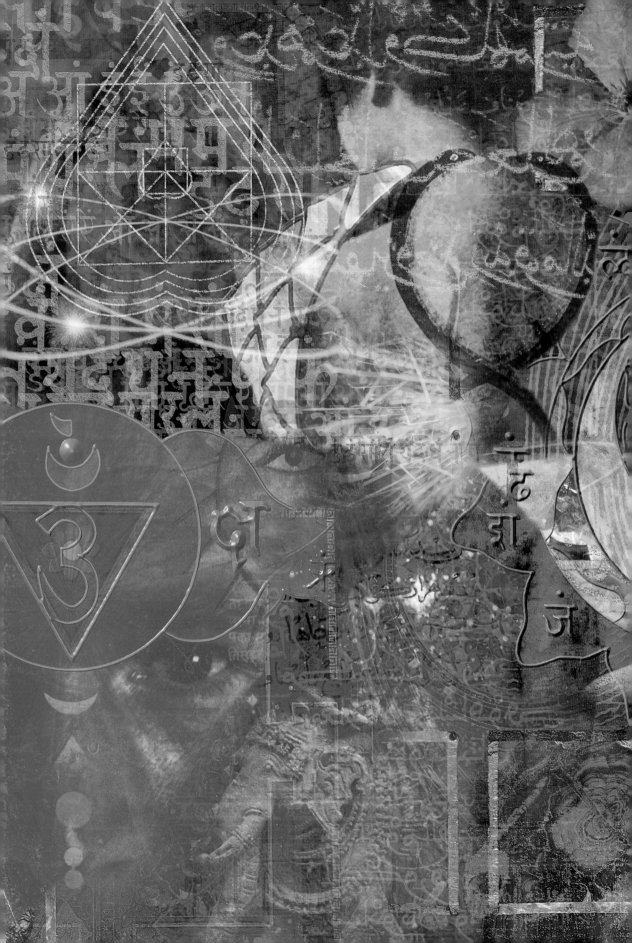

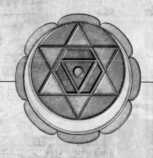

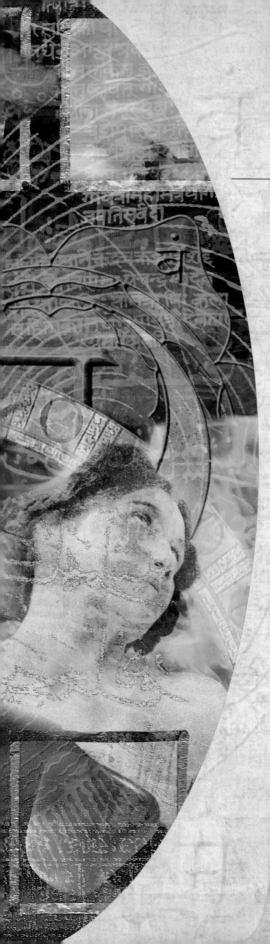

THE BOOK OF
CHAKRA
HEALING

LIZ SIMPSON

Gaia Books Limited

A GAIA ORIGINAL

Books from Gaia celebrate the vision of Gaia,
the self-sustaining living Earth, and seek to help its
readers live in greater personal and planetary harmony.

Editor	Jo Godfrey Wood
Designer	Sara Mathews
Illustrator	Mark Preston
Production	Lyn Kirby
Managing Editor	Pip Morgan
Direction	Patrick Nugent

DEDICATION

TO MARTINE, FOR WALKING
THE JOURNEY WITH ME

First published in the United Kingdom in 1999 by
Gaia Books Ltd, 66 Charlotte St, London W1P 1LR and
20 High St, Stroud, Glos GL5 1AS

ISBN 1-85675-083 3

A catalogue record of this book is available from the British Library.

Printed and bound by Kyodo, Singapore

10 9 8 7 6 5

A NOTE FROM THE AUTHOR

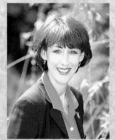 The chakras are metaphysical vortices of energy originating in the ancient Indian system of healing, which positions them in seven major centres down the body, controlling the flow of subtle energies. They symbolize the connection between the spiritual and the physical, and coincide with the body's endocrine system. When they are in balance each of the seven major chakras helps a particular part of the body to function perfectly. When unbalanced, dysfunctional, or "blocked", a whole range of mental, emotional, and physiological conditions can manifest themselves.

In this book I invite you to embark on a journey of self-discovery by working on your chakras and discovering how to balance your subtle energy system and focus on restoring your optimal physical, mental, emotional, and spiritual self. The book offers a feast of practical ways in which to work on the chakras - individually and as an interrelating system - through colours, archetypes, altar creation, physical exercises, crystal work, meditations, visualizations, daily questions, and affirmations. It is a lifelong reference guide to the chakra system, outlining each one's colour significance, key element, senses, words, glandular connections, mental functions, and dysfunctions.

Working on your chakras is a whole different way of looking at life and of exploring the self. Enjoy!

Liz Simpson

Liz Simpson, June 1998   Author photograph © Sonia Horsman

CONTENTS

▽ FOREWORD 7
▽ INTRODUCTION 8

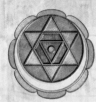

▽ THE SPIRIT OF ENERGY 12
▽ CHAKRA BALANCING 20

▽ THE ROOT (1ST) CHAKRA 35

▽ THE SACRAL (2ND) CHAKRA 49

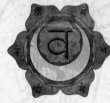

▽ THE SOLAR PLEXUS (3RD) CHAKRA 63

▽ THE HEART (4TH) CHAKRA 77

▽ THE THROAT (5TH) CHAKRA 91

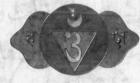

▽ THE THIRD EYE (6TH) CHAKRA 105

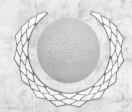

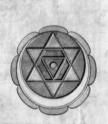

▽ THE CROWN (7TH) CHAKRA 119

▽ INTEGRATED APPROACHES 132

▽ GLOSSARY 138
▽ BIBLIOGRAPHY/RESOURCES 138-9
▽ INDEX 140

FOREWORD

Over the past few decades there has been an explosion of interest in complementary medicine. This has led to a deeper understanding of how the body functions and how energy flows through it. At the same time, people have developed a greater awareness of a more subtle energy system - the chakra system. This is like discovering a part of the anatomy that we did not know existed and being able to use it to enhance our health and well-being.

The yogis have used the chakra system for thousands of years as an integral part of holistic healing; knowing that a person's illness often first manifests itself in the chakras, before the body, mind, and emotions. Moreover, they knew that no one could be completely healed if the chakra system continued to be out of balance. Even today it is often only an advanced yogi, a healer, or "sensitive", who can "see" a blockage in a particular chakra. However, by understanding how each chakra affects a particular body function and emotion it is possible to identify where a chakra is malfunctioning. While information on the body, mind, and emotions has been presented in many books before, giving people easy access to this information, the chakras have not necessarily been presented in a user-friendly way to enable people to use this system to enhance their healing process.

Liz Simpson, in this new book, has succeeded in taking this complex subject, prone to much vague meandering, often only properly understood by yogis and healers, and simplified it, without diluting the power of chakras to heal and replenish our lives. Her brilliant use of colour through the visual medium brings the chakras to life, inspiring and enhancing our knowledge of this subject. It is only from understanding that true healing can begin, so Liz then gives us practical methods by which we can balance our own chakra systems.

This book will be of great benefit to both health care professionals and lay people and will inspire many to explore and develop their relationship with an integral part of their being - the chakras.

Teresa Hale

Teresa Hale, Founder of the Hale Clinic, London

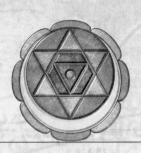

INTRODUCTION

Many people's introduction to the word "chakra" may have come, not through alternative therapy or books on Eastern approaches to well-being, but from an unexpected source. In the James Bond film, *Tomorrow Never Dies*, there is a scene in which the hero is faced with the unedifying prospect of being attacked with an ancient set of "chakra knives". These, his adversary explains, are implements of torture that can extract certain vital organs from an enemy while still alive. It is unfortunate that the concept of "chakras" - which, as you are about to discover, is so important for our health and well-being - should have been linked with such barbarism. This scene gives the impression that chakras are physically detectable in the body, which they are not. Although each chakra is closely associated with a specific organ or endocrine gland, these spinning vortices of energy are part of the subtle energy system, which forms the basis of an ancient Indian approach to healing our physical, mental, emotional, and spiritual selves.

The word chakra comes from the Sanskrit, meaning "wheel" or "disk". These moderators of subtle energy are traditionally depicted as lotus flowers, each resonating at different frequencies, corresponding to the colours of the rainbow. Although the human energy system is said to have many chakras, and new ones are being "discovered" all the time, the traditional Hindu system names seven major ones. These are positioned with the stems of each lotus flower metaphysically

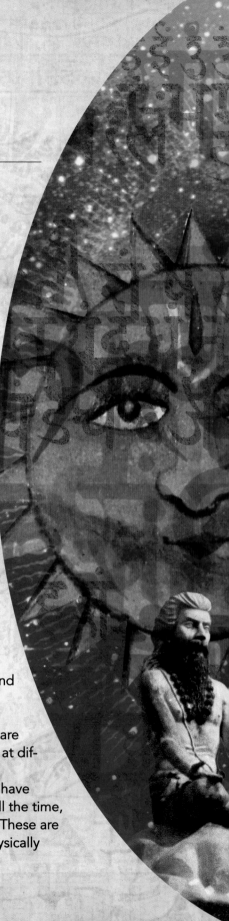

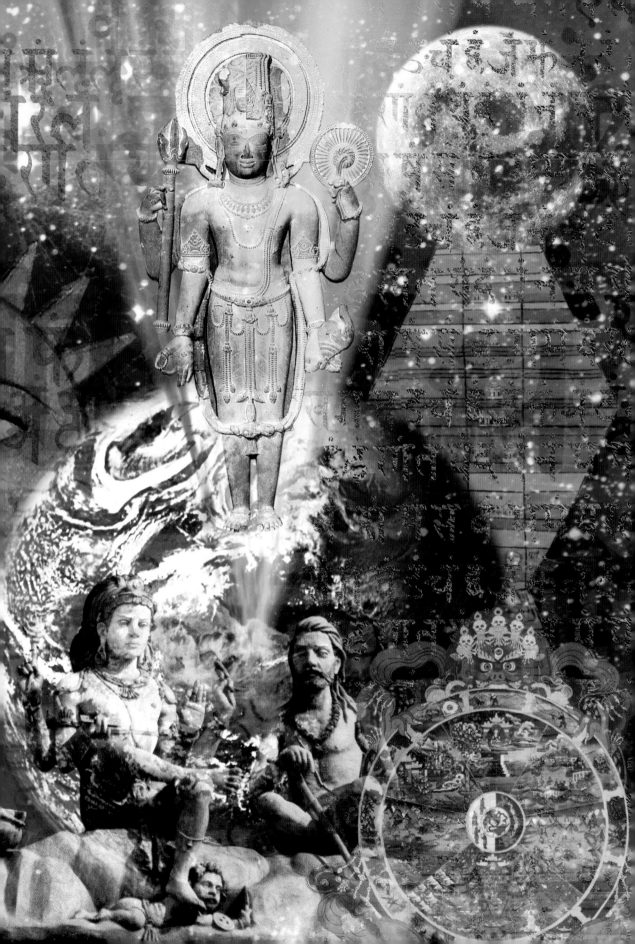

"embedded" into the spinal column, or *sushumna*, from the coccyx to the crown of the head. The chakra system has developed into a rich, valuable explanation of the holistic nature of humankind. It outlines how, in order to maintain a healthy, balanced life, we must attend not just to certain physical dysfunctions that may occur but to our emotional, intellectual, and spiritual needs as well. Each of the seven chakras deals with different parts of this bigger picture and directs us to those areas where we might be functioning out of balance.

As a different consciousness dawns at the beginning of a new millennium we are at last shaking off the confines of a purely scientific approach to life and embracing concepts that were accepted by our ancestors many thousands of years ago. Interestingly, many scientists who have become disillusioned with mainstream explanations - and the arrogance of an orthodoxy that, when it can't explain a phenomenon, dismisses it as fanciful or non-existent - are using scientific methods to explain and prove many of life's anomalies. We explore some of these new advances in the first chapter (see p.12), where we look at how the human "aura", depicted in ancient drawings as sheaths of white or golden light surrounding the bodies of saints or mystics, is simply a vibrational form of energy that - until recently - could not be recorded on scientific instruments. Our ancestors, more open-minded to things they could not see, let alone explain, had no need of such technology, since we are already equipped with an inbuilt sensor for this electromagnetic energy - our hands. As we journey together through the chakras we need only to prepare ourselves similarly - principally with an open mind. What we once took for granted as solid matter, thought to be made up of "billiard ball" atoms, is - according to quantum physicists - simply 99.9999% empty space filled with energy. The fact that we cannot physically detect our chakras or aura can be explained thus: they operate as energy fields vibrating at a rate normally undetectable by the human eye and brain. As we take this journey together, and appreciate the very real benefits that come from balancing our human energy system, we will learn to discard the need for material evidence of their existence, since personal experience and enhanced well-being will provide this for us.

The origins of the sevenfold chakra system we shall be working through is buried in the roots of Hindu culture. The earliest mention of the term "chakra" is said to come from the Vedas, the four holy books of the Hindus believed to date back before 2,500 BC, in which the god Vishnu is described as descending to Earth carrying in his four arms a chakra, a lotus flower, a club, and a conch shell. However since the time of pre-Vedic societies, in which mystics and yogis passed down their knowledge through the spoken, rather than written, word, the notion of seven "maps of consciousness" for optimum well-being goes back much further.

But why should we want to utilize a system that is rooted so far back in time? What relevance does it have to living in this day and age? In common with so many ancient practices, the chakra system takes a complete view of human experience. It integrates the natural tendency for equilibrium into the many layers that make up the self - the physical, mental, emotional, and spiritual. Chakra healing is based on the belief that in order for total well-being to take place we must act as an integrated whole. In the first chapter we learn that the chakras operate like interconnected, self-opening, valves that channel the "electrical current" of the Universal Life Force into the body. When there is a dysfunction or blockage in one part of the system it has an impact on all the other parts. Such malfunctioning can occur when the energy flowing through the chakras is either excessive or deficient. This book will help you recognize how such blockages, or dysfunctions, relate to any problems you may be experiencing and how, by using any or all of the techniques outlined in the following chapters, you can transform all aspects of your life for the better.

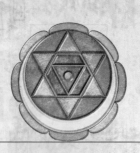

THE
SPIRIT OF ENERGY

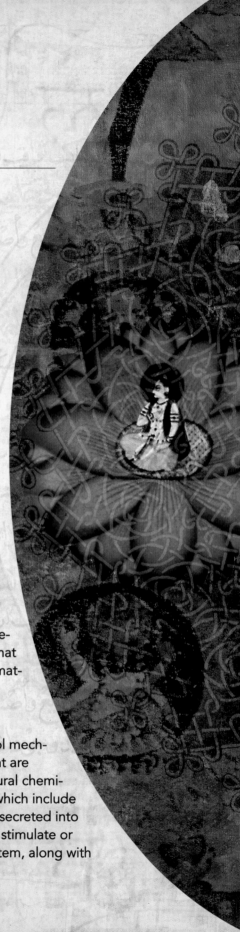

While anatomically undetectable, the seven major chakras are metaphysically linked with a number of different systems within the physical body. In this chapter we explore how the chakras bridge the visible, physical, self - in the form of the spinal cord, the autonomic nervous system, and the endocrine system - with our "subtle" body, that envelope of vibrational energy called the "aura". While orthodox medicine describes our physical system in terms of chemistry, what is now understood is that for any chemical action to take place a change in the electromagnetic energy of the body must occur. This energy emanates from the "mind" and explains the importance of the mind-body link to our physical, emotional, and mental health. The old scientific paradigm of relating to health purely in terms of the "visible" is now being superseded by an appreciation of "truths" once embraced only by mystics: that thoughts and the mind precede and affect physical matter. After all, what is thought but a form of energy?

THE ENDOCRINE SYSTEM

This system is one of the body's main physical control mechanisms. It comprises a number of ductless glands that are responsible for the production of many different natural chemicals called hormones. These chemical messengers, which include adrenalin, insulin, oestrogen, and progesterone, are secreted into the bloodstream from specific organs in the body to stimulate or inhibit certain physical processes. The endocrine system, along with

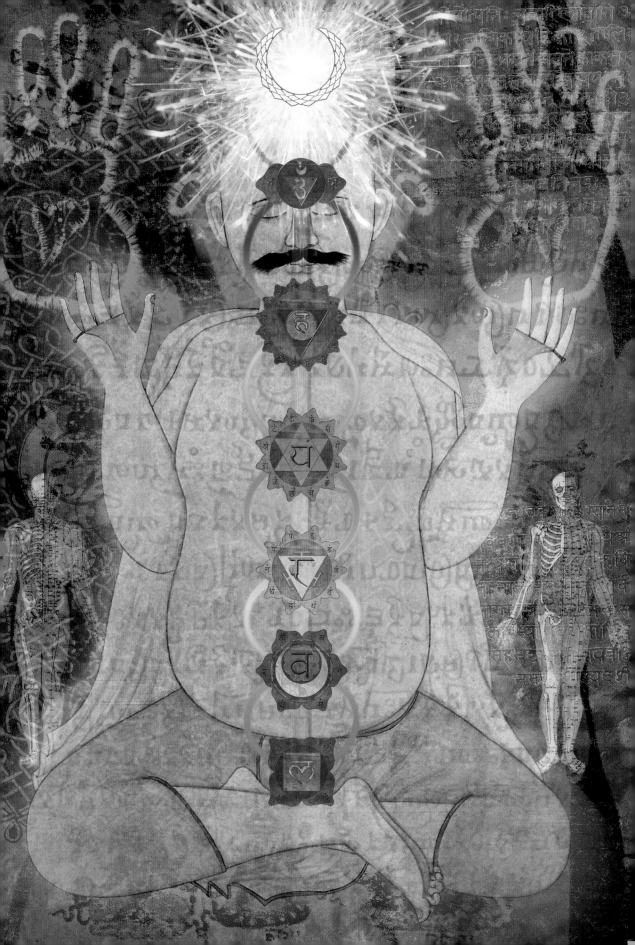

the autonomic nervous system, helps maintain the parameters needed for optimum health by adjusting levels of hormone secretion to suit special demands. In the same way that an imbalance in one chakra affects the others, the nervous and endocrine systems are functionally interconnected and any disturbance in one part can lead to a malfunction elsewhere. In order to gain a better understanding of how the endocrine system links with the chakras, let us look at each pair in turn:

ADRENALS - ROOT (1ST) CHAKRA

The adrenals are triangular-shaped glands that cap each of the kidneys. They secrete a variety of hormones including those that regulate the body's metabolism of fats, proteins, and carbohydrates and ones that control the balance of salt in our bodily fluids. These glands also produce adrenalin, the hormone essential for our primitive "fight or flight" response, from which we can determine the link between this gland and the Root Chakra's association with the issue of physical survival.

OVARIES/TESTES - SACRAL (2ND) CHAKRA

The male and female reproductive organs, or gonads, produce hormones that are responsible for the development of secondary sexual characteristics, such as the depth of voice and amount of body hair. The testes and ovaries control an individual's sexual development and maturity as well as the production of sperm in males and eggs in females. Our relationship with our own sexuality, and issues of emotional balance concerning that, is a key association of this chakra.

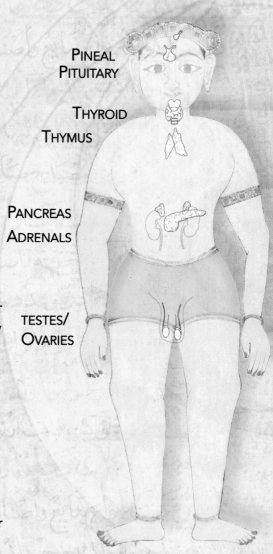

PINEAL
PITUITARY

THYROID
THYMUS

PANCREAS
ADRENALS

TESTES/
OVARIES

THE ENDOCRINE SYSTEM

The positions of the seven chakras coincide approximately with the positions of the glands in the endocrine system.

PANCREAS - SOLAR PLEXUS (3RD) CHAKRA

The pancreas lies behind the stomach and secretes a variety of
substances essential for the effective digestion of food. It also
produces insulin, which helps control the blood's sugar level.
One of the physical dysfunctions of this chakra is diabetes, a dis-
ease caused by excess sugar in the bloodstream. There is a further link with the Solar Plexus and adrenalin, which is why we
experience "butterflies in the stomach" during frightening experiences. The associated body parts of the Solar Plexus include
the digestive system and a further dysfunction of this chakra is
stomach ulcers.

THYMUS - HEART (4TH) CHAKRA

Located just above the heart, the thymus produces hormones
that stimulate general growth, particularly early in life. It also has
a purifying role in the body by stimulating the production of lymphocytes, which form part of the blood's white cells' defence
system, attacking invading organisms and providing immunity.
Scientists now recognize that auto-immune diseases, where the
immune system attacks its own proteins, mistaking them for a
foreign substance, have an emotional link and are not simply
due to physical or environmental causes.

THYROID/PARATHYROID - THROAT (5TH) CHAKRA

The thyroid gland, situated on either side of the larynx and tra-
chea in the neck, manufactures thyroxine, which controls the
body's metabolic rate - that is, how effectively it converts food
into energy. Behind this lies the parathyroid gland, which
controls the level of calcium in the bloodstream. In addition to
physical growth, these glands are also believed to affect one's
mental development. The Throat Chakra, linked with all forms of
communication, corresponds to the need for balance between
the rational, cerebral, approach and the emotional expression of
the heart.

PITUITARY - THIRD EYE (6TH) CHAKRA

The pituitary gland is located within a structure at the base of
the skull, close to the eyebrows. Once called the "master gland"

of the endocrine system, it has since been found to be controlled by hormonal substances released by the hypothalmus, a part of the brain. This vital gland influences growth, metabolism, and general body chemistry. This includes the hormone which produces contractions during labour and releases milk from the breasts during lactation. It is interesting to note this Third Eye-pituitary gland connection with birth and motherhood, a time when many women feel that their intuition, particularly with regard to their child, is at its peak.

PINEAL - CROWN (7TH) CHAKRA

The glandular connection of the Crown Chakra is the pineal gland, a pea-sized body that lies deep within the brain and was once thought to serve no useful purpose. Considered in the seventeenth century to be the seat of the soul by French philosopher, René Descartes, recent scientific research has linked this gland with the production of melatonin and regulates our internal "body clock". Melatonin is also the subject of intense scientific interest for its possible anti-ageing properties and is believed to affect the pituitary, thyroid, adrenals, and gonads - although no one yet understands how or why. Like the Crown's function within the chakra system as a whole, the pineal gland is the control centre for the effective functioning of our physical, emotional, and mental selves.

THE SUSHUMNA AND KUNDALINI RISING

In the same way that our physical body's central nervous system consists of the spinal cord leading to the brain, the energetic equivalent - the sushumna - is the vertical column within which the seven chakras are located. The parallels between these physical and metaphysical structures are striking. Whereas the function of the spinal cord is to relay impulses to and from the brain and other parts of the body, the sushumna channels energy from the Universal Life Force to and from the Crown and Root Chakras. Each chakra is rooted into the sushumna by both a front and a rear aspect. In their traditional depictions as lotus flowers, the petals of each chakra emerge from the sushumna at

KUNDALINI RISING
The serpent goddess travels from the Root Chakra to the Crown, piercing each energy centre in her path.

the front of the body, while the stems open out from the back. The stems normally remain closed and have a negative polarity, whereas the petals consecutively vibrate, rotate in a clockwise or anticlockwise direction, as well as open and close. They have a positive polarity.

The journey upward through the chakras is spoken of in terms of "Kundalini rising". Kundalini is the serpent goddess, often depicted as coiled three and a half times around the Root Chakra. According to Hindu tradition, when awakened Kundalini pierces each chakra in turn as she travels toward the crown. Once she has arrived at her destination the subject is said to have achieved enlightenment. There are many links between Kundalini and religious and cultural archetypes. In Genesis it is a serpent that leads Adam and Eve to taste from the Tree of Knowledge, thereby instigating the inner conflict between material needs and the spiritual desire to achieve higher states of consciousness. And in Egypt, the pharaohs wore serpent symbols over the Third Eye Chakra to represent godlike stature. It is the appreciation of our Higher Self - finding the God within - that is the ultimate goal of this journey through the chakras.

THE HUMAN AURA

The peoples of the ancient cultures of the East, who developed the notion of a sevenfold chakra system, knew and understood that beyond its material form the body is really a pulsating, dynamic field of energy. The concept of an "aura", depicted in early paintings as a halo of bright, multi-coloured light around the physical self, defies the laws of physics - but only as we currently understand them. Orthodox science may have been unable to measure this "spiritual" energy - in the same way that it is incapable of measuring emotional or mental energy - but there is no denying these levels of experience.

Pioneering experts in the United States and China, however, now say that the bioelectromagnetic field - or aura - of every living thing is no longer in question. Using technology developed from the NASA space programme in the United States, for example, neurophysiologist and psychologist Dr Valerie V. Hunt has scientifically verified that there are two primary electrical systems in the physical body. The first is the alternating electrical current of the nervous system and brain which governs our muscles, hormones, and physical sensations. The second is a continuous, electromagnetic radiation coming off our atoms which allows for an energy exchange between individuals and their environment.

Each person's unique energy field - said to surround them like an envelope - is accessed from a universal pool known as the Universal Life Force, "prana", or "chi" (or Qi). This pool of energy is drawn into the body through each of the chakras and is transformed by them into a particular quality, dominant sense, and emotional correlate. The chakras act like a series of valves in a system connecting a water tap to a garden hose. Once the tap is turned on, the water should flow smoothly through the system. But if there is a kink in the hose (analogous to a blockage of energy) or if any of the valves are too open or too closed, this affects the proper functioning of the whole unit.

Experts now believe that the field of radiation, which we call the aura, in combination with our DNA, makes up our combined genetic material. It seems that while the passive DNA preserves our unique genetic code, the transmitting bioelectromagnetic field is able to modify it. Ancient healers believed that the aura holds the key to a person's physical, mental, emotional, and spiritual states. Scientists working in the field of energy medicine back this up, saying that this vibrating energy field, banded in layers around the physical body like a set of Russian dolls, is similar to the magnetic tape of a tape recorder which stores coded information about our past, present, and future health. And that by maintaining an open and smooth flowing channel of energy through our chakras, by freeing ourselves of the mental or emotional traumas that can cause blockages, we can pre-empt the onset of physical dis-ease. The next chapter (see p.20) outlines how you can use the information in the rest of this book to re-balance your own chakra system.

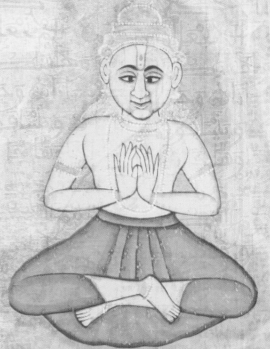

A HEALTHY AURA
A smooth, steady flow of energy through the chakra system ensures a healthy aura, in turn indicating a body clear from dis-ease.

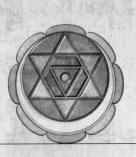

CHAKRA
BALANCING

I have already used the analogy of a hose and water
to illustrate how the chakras function as a complete
system (see p.18). Another way to demonstrate
their inter-connectedness is to think of them as individual gears in an interconnecting structure of
cogged wheels (see p.22). Imagine what would
happen if one of these wheels revolved too fast or
too slowly in comparison with the others. The
entire system would become unbalanced and
would have to be re-aligned before it could work
properly again. Similarly, our chakras become dysfunctional, not only through being too open but
also by vibrating, or "spinning", sluggishly because
of some emotionally based blockage - usually rooted
in childhood. Once you have identified which
dysfunctions relate to your particular life challenges, it
will be easier to home in on those chakras you need to
pay particular attention to, and the methods you can
use to bring them back into equilibrium. However,
always remember to think of the chakra system in its
entirety and how each one works in harmony with the others, to bring you to a complete sense of well-being. Each
chakra operates at a unique, optimum frequency which
determines its colours and its other characteristics. However,
this frequency can be detrimentally affected through receiving
too much or too little energy from the Universal Life Force. There
are various schools of thought as to why such dysfunctions occur.
Some say they stem from Karmic patterning - that is, we come into
this life with a certain set of life challenges factored in to our chakras.

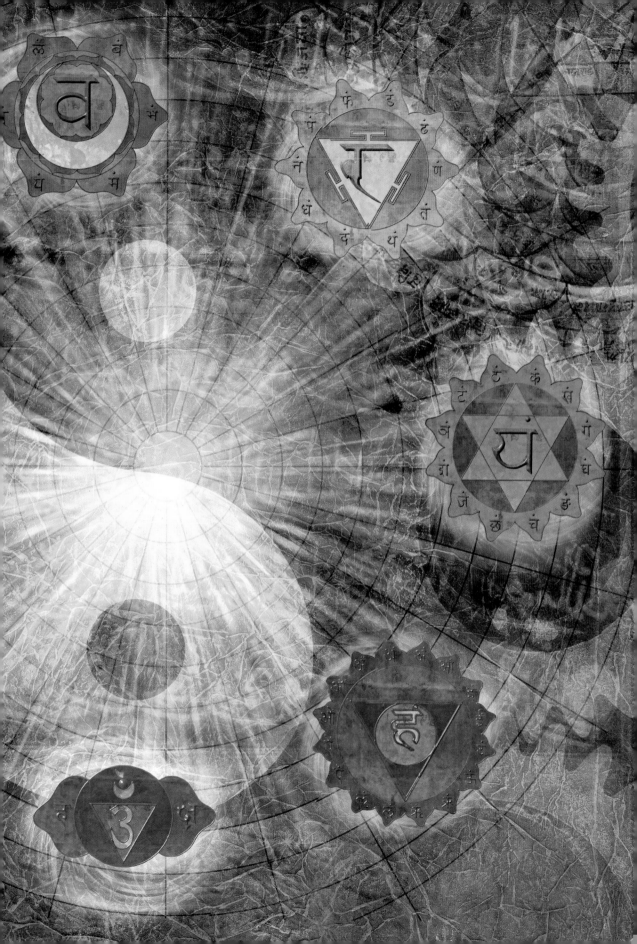

This "prior programming" determines our subsequent attitudes and behaviours. Similarly, many therapists believe that the deficient or excessive energy patterning of our chakras stems from our childhood and cultural experiences. They say that one of the ways in which we cope with certain repeating situations is to try and protect ourselves by closing down the relevant chakra. So, if we are criticized or neglected constantly in our early years, when we lack the inner resources or mental capacity to cope, we begin to feel inadequate and unlovable. This emotional insecurity becomes confused with our basic survival needs and subconsciously we close down the chakra as a defence mechanism. Whichever explanation resonates with you, never forget that we operate, in our personal lives, in a "free will zone". We have a choice as to whether we accept or attempt to change the challenging situations which our predispositions cause us to attract in life. Knowledge is power.

(See the Chakra Correspondences in each chakra chapter to assess your dysfunctions: Root pp.36-7; Sacral pp.50-1; Solar Plexus pp.64-5; Heart pp.78-9; Throat pp.92-3; Third Eye pp.106-7; Crown pp.120-1.)

SEVEN WAYS TO BALANCE YOUR CHAKRAS

In the same way that no one alternative health approach suits everybody, and you may need to experience several before you discover the one that works best for you, there are various different ways of balancing your chakras. This chapter explains the menu of approaches outlined in the following chakra chapters. Try them all; there is bound to be one that resonates with you and becomes your favourite. However, it is important to sample the others, too. Even if you feel pre-disposed to focusing on the yoga-based exercises, for example, there may be occasions when it is inconvenient to practise them for a few days. At such times it may be helpful to exercise your mind by reflecting on the archetypes linked with the chakras, doing some meditation or guided visualizations, or keeping a daily questions journal.

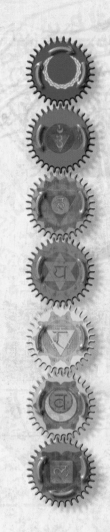

INTERCONNECTING WHEELS
When all seven chakras are spinning in harmony, at the same speed, the system runs smoothly, as a single mechanism.

1. ARCHETYPES

These are universal themes, or models, of the "human condition". Illustrated through myths, fairy stories, and even modern films, they provide us with an understanding of our emotional experiences - both what we are and what we would like to become. Through these "life dramas" we learn about the different values that underpin our attitudes, beliefs, and behaviours. Archetypal storytelling polarizes the choices we make in tackling life's challenges; whether to opt for courage or cowardice, patience or impetuousness, thought or action. Archetypes are far more "black and white" than real life is, so that we can see more clearly the choices on offer. However, there are times when both functional and dysfunctional archetypes are valuable for spiritual growth. While we may choose to suppress our "dark side" we should accept that we can never totally eradicate it. Our mission toward self-ownership and enlightenment includes acknowledging those parts of ourselves that we may not instinctively like or admire; our free will is strengthened from never letting them have total power over us.

By identifying the patterns we may have embedded into our neural pathways and which are outwardly projected as particular behaviours, we can choose to discard those that no longer serve us. There are both dysfunctional and functional archetypes associated with each chakra. Understanding how these influence our lives can help us take up the reins of the emotional challenges that face us daily in order that we can choose to take a different direction and move on to a new stage of development.

(See the Archetype pages in each chakra chapter: Root pp.38-9; Sacral pp.52-3; Solar Plexus pp.66-7; Heart pp.80-1; Throat pp.94-5; Third Eye pp.108-9; Crown pp.122-3.)

2. Altars

So much of the work we do on ourselves - such as meditation, visualization, and other forms of introspection - is intangible, so it is good to have something physical to concentrate on and to act as a focal point for mental work. An "altar" is your own sacred space; somewhere you can create a celebration, or even a ritual, for the chakra you choose to work on. Centuries ago our ancestors realized that there was great psychological comfort to be gained from rituals, which is why institutions from religions, nations, and workplaces - even the way we lay the table before family meals - involve ritualized practices. In an age when routine and ritual seem to be fading from our lives, creating a personal altar - no matter how small - offers valuable grounding and a chance to express yourself creatively.

Through the association with colour and the personal selection of items inspired by the relevant chart of correspondences, creating an altar will help you become more mindful of the issues and challenges concerning the particular chakra you are currently working on. Once you have got into the habit of attending to your altar daily - whether to clean or reorganize it, or change some of the objects - it will be much easier to include a set amount of time for meditative thought. Remember that this is *your* sacred space and you should only include items that have meaning and offer inspiration for you. The altars shown in this book are case study examples, for inspiration only. It can be a valuable exercise to meditate on what you might like to include before you start - allowing your intuitive self to guide you. Refer back to the Correspondence charts in each chakra chapter for ideas on what to include. Experiment with the layout and if one of the items irritates or upsets you, or is less than inspiring, remove it.

(See the Altar pages in each chakra chapter: Root pp.40-1; Sacral pp.54-5; Solar Plexus pp.68-9; Heart pp.82-3; Throat pp.96-7; Third Eye pp.110-11; Crown pp.124-5.)

3. Physical Exercises

With the exception of the Third Eye, which, because of its nature, responds to mental discipline, there are physical exercises suggested for each chakra. These are largely based on yoga movements which have been developed down the ages as a way of embracing physical stimulation, the necessary mental focus for proper breathing, and meditative repose to boost the spirit. Yoga's link with the chakras will come as no surprise when you learn that the origins of both stem from the Hindu scriptures - the Vedas.

As a safe discipline, which anyone can practise, yoga postures help to stretch and tone the body both internally and externally. These exercises will help to release any physical and mental tension contributing to the improper functioning of your chakras. Even those sceptical of the metaphysical benefits of practising yoga should know that medical research into its beneficial effects include studies that have shown a reduction in high blood pressure, a significant increase in lung capacity and respiration, improved ability to resist stress, as well as relief from conditions such as arthritis, asthma, chronic fatigue, and heart problems. When we are physically well it is much easier to deal with mental and emotional challenges, and yoga is one valuable way of achieving that total well-being.

(See the Exercise pages in each chakra chapter: Root pp.42-3; Sacral pp.56-7; Solar Plexus pp.70-1; Heart pp.84-5; Throat pp.98-9; Third Eye pp.112-13; Crown pp.126-7.)

Before You Start Physical Exercises

▽ Do not exercise straight after a heavy meal. Wait at least 4 hours, and 2 hours after a snack.

▽ Go to the bathroom before you start.

▽ Wear loose-fitting clothes and remove your shoes.

▽ Use a non-slip mat or heavy blanket.

▽ Don't strain your body to achieve any of the positions.

▽ Spend a few minutes practising your breathing beforehand. Inhale through the nose and out through the mouth. Breathe slowly and smoothly as you work through the movements.

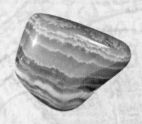

4. CRYSTAL HEALING

The chakras are vortices of energy through which the Universal Life Force is channelled and transmitted. They resonate at different frequencies, which we, in the physical dimension, associate with different colours. Crystals work on the same principle. They oscillate to a natural healing frequency that is activated by the power of the mind. This is achieved by techniques such as meditation and visualization. Crystals are therefore compatible tools with which to harmonize and balance the chakras. They can help you tap in to your natural self-healing abilities, promoting optimum physical, mental, and spiritual well-being.

All you need to do to unlock this vibrational healing potential is to focus your mental energy on crystals positioned on or near the relevant chakra. The examples found in each of the chakra chapters suggest which colours or specific crystals to use. Through the power of intention - yours or your therapist's - the appropriate healing energy from the Universal Life Force is channelled through the crystal. This energy becomes amplified through the unique molecular structure of natural crystals and helps to stimulate, balance, or relax the chakra frequencies.

The crystal body layouts for each chakra demonstrate a selection of crystals and suggested placements for each chakra, though these are case study examples so should not be copied slavishly. In two cases the individuals involved chose single crystals rather than multi-crystal layouts (Heart and Third Eye Chakras). You will be guided toward the most effective layout for your needs by the individual chart of correspondences for each chakra. There you will find an outline of the associated physical and emotional dysfunctions. But be advised to always take expert advice on any severe medical condition before substituting treatment for an alternative approach such as crystal healing.

(See the Crystal pages in each chakra chapter: Root pp.44-5; Sacral pp.58-9; Solar Plexus pp.72-3; Heart pp.86-7; Throat pp.100-1; Third Eye pp.114-15; Crown pp.128-9.)

CHOOSING CRYSTALS

Check the crystals which relate to each chakra (see chakra chapters). If you need to buy them, select the appropriate colour and use your intuition to choose the right crystals for your specific needs. Once cleansed and tuned, close your eyes and, focusing on the relevant chakra, run your hand over the crystals. Pick out the ones that feel "right". This sense may even be physical and involve a tingling sensation.

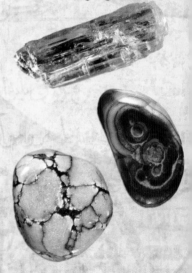

USING CRYSTALS

Lie down and position the crystals within easy reach. Use a meditation exercise to tune in to the chakra you are working on and become aware of the wheel- or flower-like structure. Position the crystal(s) on or near the chakra. Follow a meditation (see individual chakras) to allow the vibrations from the crystal to energize the chakra. Afterwards, ease yourself back to normal consciousness.

CLEANSING CRYSTALS

This is a spiritual ritual by which inappropriate energies can be neutralized and crystals re-energized. Choose one of the following methods:

▽ Hold them under running water, visualizing a beautiful waterfall or waves on a beach.

▽ Ring a bell over them.

▽ Leave them in the sun for 24 hours.

▽ Smudge them by burning dried herbs and wafting smoke over them.

▽ Use an Amethyst bed to cleanse a group of crystals at once.

▽ Hold your crystals and imagine bright white light pouring down from your Crown, washing away all negativity.

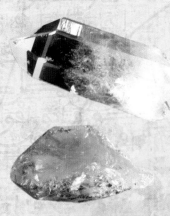

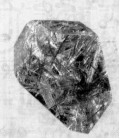

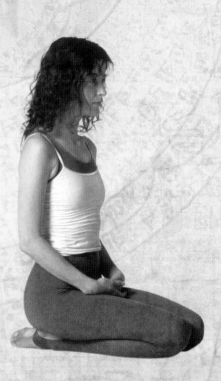

TUNING

When you cleanse crystals you "switch them on", like turning on a radio. But to receive a "broadcast" you must tune the dial to the correct station. Also the "wavelength" you choose when tuning depends on your purpose. Say: "I intend this crystal to be an effective tool for healing/meditation/dream interpretation, etc."

5. MEDITATION

Psychologists have discovered that the brain cannot differentiate between what is real and what is realistically imagined. There are many benefits to be derived from taking part in regular meditations and guided visualizations:

▽ *They offer a rare opportunity to be still and silent and able to hear that "still, small voice" of inner wisdom and intuition.*

▽ *Calming the mind automatically calms the body, helping to reduce stress and giving the physical self the opportunity to rebalance.*

▽ *When the mind is calm you can sense where physical pain originates and "feel" where a particular chakra might be out of balance.*

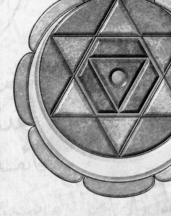

▽ *Our minds are mental sports fields and theatre stages on which we can "play out" scenarios, which, in real life, might be dangerous. By imagining different options we can safely check out the effects of each and come to the right conclusion on which to take action.*

▽ *Few of us, as adults, allow our imagination full rein. Playing "make believe" is vital for emotional development - even for "grownups".*

▽ *Everything we see or touch started as a thought. Whatever you can think, you can create, and meditations and visualizations ensure that your resulting creations contribute to your complete well-being.*

6. DAILY QUESTIONS

Knowledge is power. The more we understand ourselves the better equipped we are to make positive changes in our lives. The questions that relate to each chakra's life challenge will help you unpick the ways in which you sabotage your happiness and well-being with dysfunctional attitudes and behaviours. They will also help you determine how to bring about those physical, mental, emotional, and spiritual changes which will assist the more effective functioning of your chakras.

Keeping a journal is vital for self-development. We have so many thoughts each day it is difficult to keep pace with them and virtually impossible - unless we write them down - to ascertain the patterns that underpin our attitudes to life. As you make your journey through the chakras your journal will help you chart progress and motivate you toward even greater personal development. Looking back in days, months, or even years, to come, you will find the truth in Charlie Chaplin's assertion that: "Life is a tragedy when seen close-up, but a comedy in long-shot."

Acquire a beautifully bound notebook and write your thoughts nightly for the next three weeks. That's the length of time we need to perform a new behaviour in order to turn it into a habit. Don't worry about how much or how little you write. The important thing is to select a question that resonates with you and the particular challenge you are facing at this time, and let your consciousness lead you to the answer.

7. AFFIRMATIONS

Imagine a field of grass across which you must walk each day. Every time you take the same route you crush the grass underfoot until, eventually, a distinct pathway appears. Similarly, every time you have a particular thought a neural pathway is created in the brain - a weak link at first, but one which gets stronger the more times the same thought is brought to mind. That is why it is so difficult to break habitual patterns of thinking; they have become so embedded in our brain that we need to create another, more compelling, "pathway" to compete with them. This is what we do when we say affirmations. These are positive sentences which "tell" our brain that we are choosing to think differently about a particular life challenge. And just like the grass analogy, the more we tread the same path - that is, the more we speak and think these beneficial, optimistic messages to ourselves - the greater our chances of changing old, inappropriate, patterns of thought and behaviour.

(See Meditation, Daily Questions, Affirmations pages in each chakra chapter: Root pp.46-7; Sacral pp.60-1; Solar Plexus pp.74-5; Heart pp.88-9; Throat pp.102-3; Third Eye pp.116-17; Crown pp.130-1.)

THE MAIN CHART OF CORRESPONDENCES

Chakra & Location	Sanskrit Name & Meaning	Associated Colour	Main Issue
Crown (7th) Top of head	*Sahasrara* Thousandfold	Violet, gold, white	Spirituality
Third Eye (6th) Above & between eyebrows	*Ajna* To perceive, to know	Indigo	Intuition, Wisdom
Throat (5th) Centrally, at base of neck	*Vishuddha* Purification	Blue	Communication, Self-expression
Heart (4th) Centre of chest	*Anahata* Unstruck	Green/pink	Love & Relationships
Solar Plexus (3rd) Between navel & base of sternum	*Manipura* Lustrous gem	Yellow	Personal power, Self will
Sacral (2nd) Lower abdomen, between navel & genitals	*Svadhisthana* Sweetness	Orange	Emotional balance/ Sexuality
Root (1st) Between anus & genitals	*Muladhara* Root or Support	Red	Survival/ Physical needs

Glandular Connection	Associated Body Parts	Element & Ruling Planet	Astrological Associations	Associated Sense
Pineal	Upper skull, cerebral cortex, skin	Thought/cosmic energy Uranus	Aquarius	Beyond Self
Pituitary	Eyes, base of skull	Light/Telepathic energy Neptune, Jupiter	Sagittarius, Pisces	Sixth sense
Thyroid, Parathyroid	Mouth, throat, ears	Ether Mercury	Gemini, Virgo	Sound/hearing
Thymus	Heart & chest, lungs, circulation	Air Venus	Libra, Taurus	Touch
Pancreas	Digestive system, muscles	Fire Mars & Sun	Aries, Leo	Sight
Ovaries, Testes	Sex organs, bladder, prostate, womb	Water Pluto	Cancer, Scorpio	Taste
Adrenals	Bones, skeletal structure	Earth Saturn	Capricorn	Smell

(Continued overleaf)

THE MAIN CHART OF CORRESPONDENCES (CONTINUED)

Chakra & Location	Fragrances, Incense/Oils	Crystals	Animals & Archetypes
Crown (7th) Top of head	Lavender, Frankincense, Rosewood	Amethyst, Clear quartz, Diamond	(None) Guru/ Egocentric
Third Eye (6th) Above & between eyebrows	Hyacinth, Violet, Rose geranium	Amethyst, Fluorite, Azurite	(None) Psychic/ Rationalist
Throat (5th) Centrally, at base of neck	Chamomile, Myrrh	Lapis lazuli, Turquoise, Aquamarine	Elephant, bull Communicator/ Masked Self
Heart (4th) Centre of chest	Rose, Bergamot, Melissa	Watermelon tourmaline, Rose quartz, Emerald	Gazelle/ antelope Lover/ Performer
Solar Plexus (3rd) Between navel & base of sternum	Vetivert, Ylang ylang, Bergamot	Aventurine quartz, Sunstone, Yellow citrine	Ram Spiritual Warrior/Drudge
Sacral (2nd) Lower abdomen, between navel & genitals	Jasmine, Rose, Sandalwood	Citrine, Carnelian, Golden topaz	Fish-tailed Alligator Sovereign/ Martyr
Root (1st) Between anus & genitals	Cedarwood, Myrrh, Patchouli	Hematite, Tiger's eye, Bloodstone	Elephant Earth Mother/ Victim

Physical Dysfunctions	Emotional Dysfunctions	Sacramental Association	Foods	Developmental Age & Life Lesson
Sensitivity to pollutants, chronic exhaustion, epilepsy, Alzheimer's	Depression, obsessional thinking, confusion	Extreme Unction	(None) Fasting	(N/A) Selflessness
Headaches, poor vision, neurological disturbances, glaucoma	Nightmares, learning difficulties, hallucinations	Ordination	(None)	(N/A) Emotional intelligence
Sore throats, neckache, thyroid problems, tinnitus, asthma	Perfectionism, inability to express emotions, blocked creativity	Confession	Fruit	28-35 yrs Personal expression
Shallow breathing, high blood pressure, heart disease, cancer	Fears about betrayal, co-dependent, melancholic	Marriage	Vegetables	21-28 yrs Forgiveness & compassion
Stomach ulcers, digestive problems, chronic fatigue, allergies, diabetes	Oversensitive to criticism, need to be in control, low self-esteem	Confirmation	Complex carbohydrates	14-21 yrs Self-esteem/ self-confidence
Impotence, frigidity, bladder & prostate problems, lower back pain	Unbalanced sex drive, emotional instability, feelings of isolation	Communion	Liquids	8-14 yrs Challenging motivations based on social conditioning
Osteoarthritis	Mental lethargy, "spaciness", incapable of inner stillness	Baptism	Proteins, meats	1-8 yrs Standing up for oneself

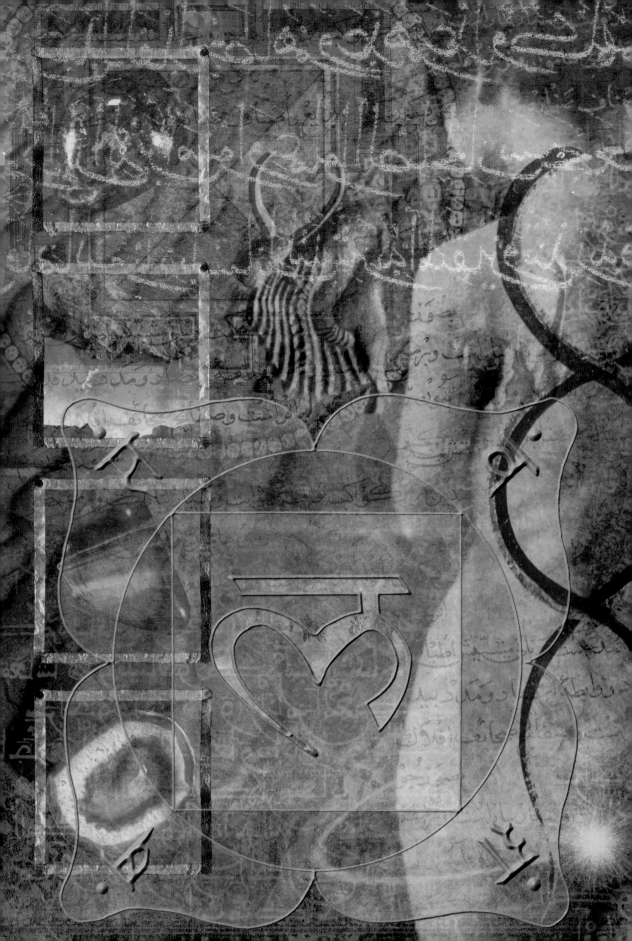

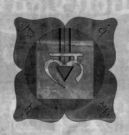

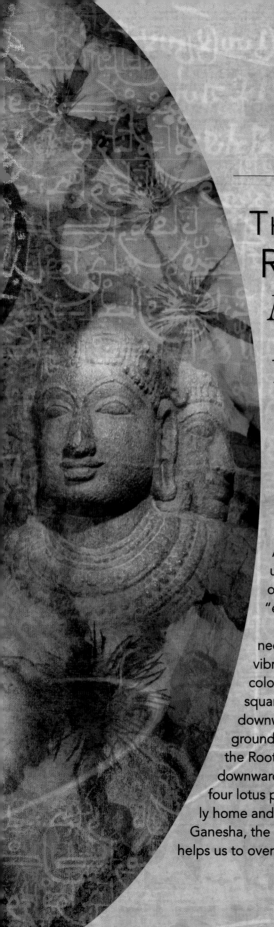

THE
ROOT CHAKRA
MULADHARA

The journey through the chakras begins with the Root (First) Chakra. Its Sanskrit name, *Muladhara*, meaning "root" or "support", is depicted as a four-petalled lotus flower encompassing a downward-pointing triangle, set within a square. In more complex versions of the symbol the Goddess Kundalini – a coiled snake wrapped around a phallus, or *lingam*, represents male sexuality. Female sexuality is located primarily in the Sacral (Second) Chakra. According to Hindu tradition, Kundalini moves upward through the chakras, awakening each one in turn, until she reaches the Crown, when "enlightenment" is achieved.

The Root Chakra is concerned with physical needs and basic human survival. It has the lowest vibrational rate of all the chakras, resonating to the colour red. The element Earth is represented by the square, or *yantra*, and the inverted triangle denotes downward movement of energy, which keeps us grounded to the Earth. And so there is a link between the Root Chakra and gravity, which constantly pulls us downward, connecting us to our material existence. The four lotus petals symbolize the four elements of our earthly home and the deity commonly associated with it is Ganesha, the elephant-headed god, which Hindus believe helps us to overcome obstacles.

ROOT CHAKRA CORRESPONDENCES

This chart for the Root (First) Chakra identifies all the associations and symbolisms linked with this particular chakra. As such it provides a "ready reference" of inspirations to use when you carry out practical exercises such as assembling your altar arrangements (see pp.40-1) or choosing appropriate stones for crystal work (see pp.44-5). This chart will also help you with the various images you will need when composing your own meditations and visualizations. Incorporate as many of these symbols and themes as you feel is appropriate to your needs.

By reacquainting yourself regularly with this chakra chart as a prelude to the section on the Root Chakra, you will help to keep your mind focused on related issues, including an awareness of your physical body and your survival needs through diet, exercise, and interactions with the "tribe", or group identity.

To make your chakra journey successful and enjoyable you should prepare yourself by attending to certain practical requirements (see pp.25 and 45). Mastering the Root Chakra helps you grasp the importance of a fit, healthy body as you travel upward through higher and higher levels of consciousness.

CHAKRA CHARACTERISTICS

See which of the following characteristics of excessive ("too open"), deficient ("blocked"), and balanced chakra energy you can relate to - and then determine (should you choose) to take the necessary action, using the tools and techniques outlined in this chapter.

Too open (chakra spins too fast) - bullying, overly materialistic, self-centred, engages in physical foolhardiness
Blocked (chakra spins sluggishly or not at all) - emotionally needy, low self-esteem, self-destructive behaviour, fearful
Balanced (chakra maintains equilibrium and spins at correct vibrational speed) - demonstrates self-mastery, high physical energy, grounded, healthy

THE ROOT CHAKRA

Sanskrit Name
Muladhara

Meaning
Root or Support

Location
Base of spine, between anus & genitals

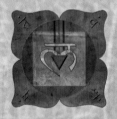

Symbol
Four red petals, around a square containing downward-pointing triangle.

Associated Colour
Red

Element
Earth

Ruling Planet
Saturn

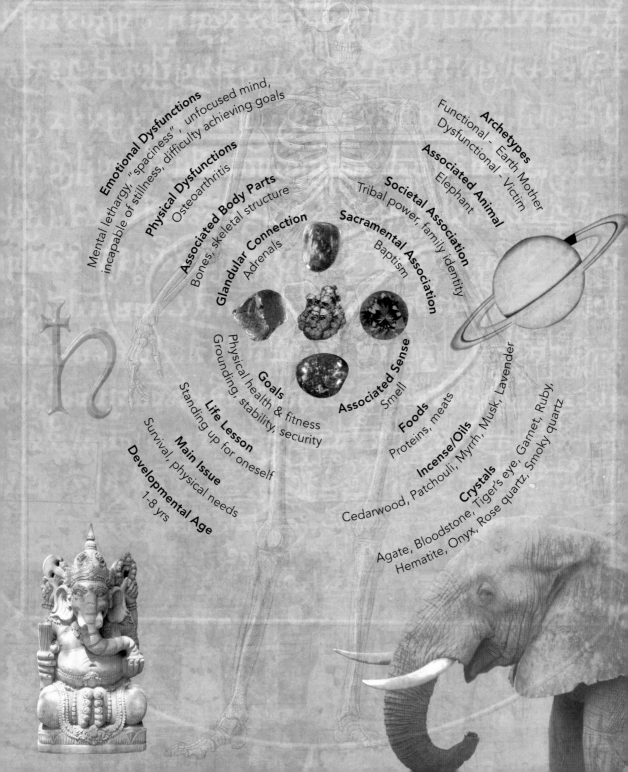

Emotional Dysfunctions
Mental lethargy, "spaciness", unfocused mind, incapable of stillness, difficulty achieving goals

Physical Dysfunctions
Osteoarthritis

Associated Body Parts
Bones, skeletal structure

Glandular Connection
Adrenals

Goals
Physical health & fitness

Life Lesson
Standing up for oneself

Main Issue
Survival, physical needs

Developmental Age
1-8 yrs

Sacramental Association
Baptism

Societal Association
Tribal power, family identity

Associated Animal
Elephant

Archetypes
Functional - Earth Mother
Dysfunctional - Victim

Associated Sense
Smell

Foods
Proteins, meats

Incense/Oils
Cedarwood, Patchouli, Myrrh, Musk, Lavender

Crystals
Agate, Bloodstone, Tiger's eye, Garnet, Ruby, Hematite, Onyx, Rose quartz, Smoky quartz

Grounding, stability, security

ARCHETYPES: ROOT CHAKRA

The Root (First) Chakra is associated with physical security. Our earliest experiences, including the extent to which our basic needs were met, or not, when infants, are recorded and stored there - like a message on a magnetic tape. Whether we are conscious of it or not, our emotional security comes from a sense of belonging to a group. This fundamental aspect of our psychological well-being relates to the Root Chakra.

"Tribal" power may not seem to apply to today's lifestyles, when we shop for provisions rather than relying on the group to hunt or gather. But most of us can acknowledge the good feelings engendered by being part of a family, having shared interests with friends, or being a member of a club. When we explore this concept of "the tribe", or the "mass mind", we can see how many of our beliefs, values, attitudes, and behaviours stem from fitting in, or not fitting in, with such groups. We may not consciously be aware of how much, such as being fed by our mother as a baby (see right).

The archetypes associated with the Root Chakra are the Earth Mother and the Victim. They represent two sides of the same coin - the positive face and our darker side. Dysfunctional Victims are increasingly commonplace in our society as people look for others to blame for their problems. If you feel you are a Victim you allow yourself to become vulnerable, needy, and hence ungrounded, because you regard every disappointment, separation, or loss as something that you cannot control or change. Subconsciously you may still consider yourself to be the baby who can't get up and feed itself and so has to rely on others. Only by recognizing that you have the power to provide everything you need for yourself can you reframe your experiences into opportunities for self-sufficiency, strength, and emotional wholeness. Changing this negative archetype involves taking personal responsibility for your life, acknowledging that you have choices and deserve the best that life has to offer.

Conversely, the functional side of this archetype is the Earth Mother, universally associated with nourishment,

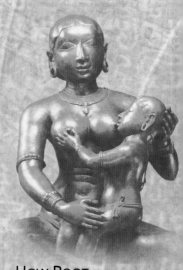

HOW ROOT ARCHETYPES MAY DEVELOP

Psychologists say that babies fed "on demand" learn to trust that their needs will be met. If this is reinforced, these individuals go through life expecting the same and are rarely disappointed. Babies left to cry learn to distrust and expect disappointments, believing that they do not deserve their needs to be met. This can affect how they conduct relationships later on in life.

caring, and unconditional love. By recognizing the Earth Mother within you (regardless of gender) you acknowledge that you are capable of providing all the physical and emotional security you need for yourself, by yourself. You can begin to develop this ability in a practical way by attending to your inner child's needs, by keeping your home environment safe and comforting, by treating yourself in a motherly way from time to time, and affirming that there is nothing you cannot accomplish, either single-handedly or by asking others for help.

THE EARTH MOTHER

This archetype is associated with nourishment, caring, and unconditional love. Attending to one's inner child by mothering oneself and keeping safe and comforted, nurtures this positive archetype.

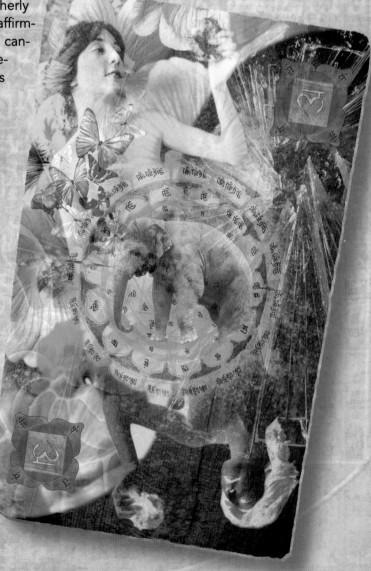

THE VICTIM

Victims let themselves become vulnerable, needy, and ungrounded. They feel that they cannot exert influence, effect change, or take control of situations.

By trying out the meditation, daily questions, and affirmations on pages 46-7 you will be able to explore the themes of Earth Mother and Victim to help you take control of your life.

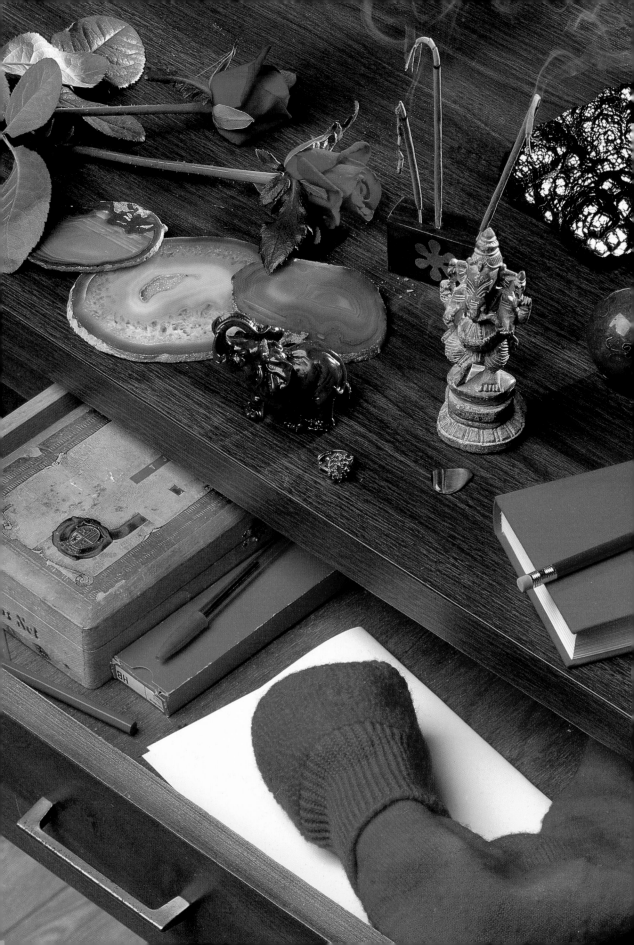

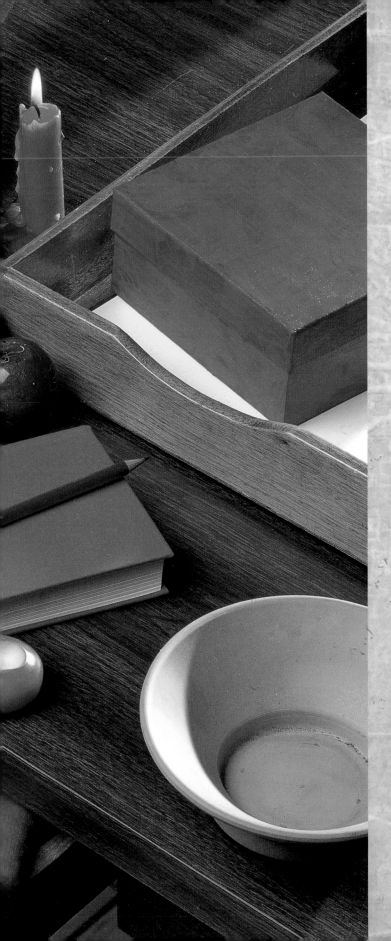

ALTAR: ROOT CHAKRA

Peter had recently lost his domineering mother. Months after her funeral he realized that he'd always espoused her beliefs unquestioningly. By allowing her to dominate way beyond childhood he had failed to assume responsibility for his own life. Now he had to start mothering himself and providing for his own needs. He also recognized how stagnant his life was, particularly his inability to overcome recurrent minor illnesses. Because of "poor health" he'd held only menial jobs and had never realized his full potential.

This altar helped focus his energies on changing his diet to tackle chronic constipation and obesity and prompted him to make the effort to socialize and "get back to the Earth" by joining a rambling club.

▽ Red, iron Baoding balls
▽ Roses - his favourite flowers
▽ Carved, dark wood elephant
▽ Grounding crystals: Agate, Hematite, and Tiger's eye
▽ Cedarwood incense sticks
▽ Model of Ganesha, the elephant-headed god linked with starting new ventures
▽ Red notebook for recording dietary progress
▽ His mother's ruby ring
▽ Red box containing details of hobby groups and societies
▽ A pair of red walking socks
▽ Red candles to light during meditations
▽ An earthenware pot to represent "grounding"

This altar is Peter's attempt to work on the Root Chakra. It is a case study, for inspiration. Choose objects of personal significance to you.

EXERCISE: ROOT CHAKRA

This exercise is a variation on one known in yoga as the "bridge" pose, or *setu bandhasara*. Its simplicity allows you to focus mentally on becoming more grounded, as well as stimulating the energy flow in the Root Chakra.

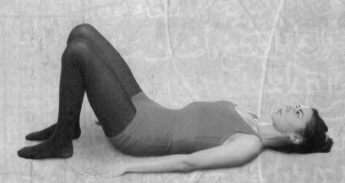

1. Lie on the floor with your arms relaxed by your sides, knees bent, and the soles of your feet a shoulder-width apart. Take a deep breath and press your lower back into the floor as you breathe out.

2. With the outbreath, push your buttocks upward, starting at the lower thigh, then moving upward toward the groin and pelvis. The way to get the correct position is to imagine a piece of string connected to your tailbone being pulled toward the ceiling. Only go as far as is comfortable, particularly if you have back problems. Make sure your lower legs are vertical.

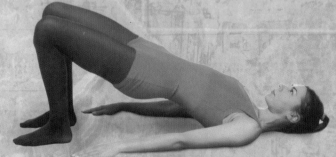

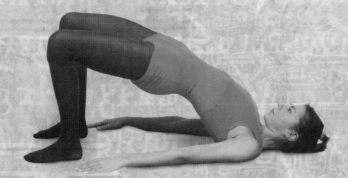

3. Continue pushing upward as long as it feels comfortable, contracting your buttock muscles to protect your lower back.

4. Come back down slowly, bringing the upper back down to the floor first, followed eventually by the tailbone. Slide your arms outward to improve your balance. Allow yourself to rest for a few minutes, feeling your whole body connect with the Earth.

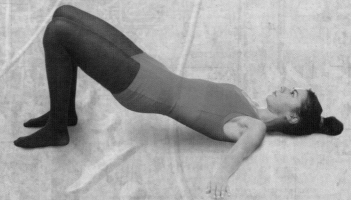

Key Crystals: Root Chakra

The Root Chakra, linked with the material world, is connected with the Earth. It stresses the importance of being grounded in the here and now. Crystals which correspond to "earthy" colours - such as brown, grey, black, and red - are all suitable for this chakra. These suggestions will help ground and centre you, in addition to their individual uses. (See also pp.26-7 for information on Crystal Healing.)

Bloodstone

A dark-green Quartz, spotted with flecks of iron oxide resembling drops of blood, this "stone of courage" helps alleviate anxieties that can unbalance the body. It is said to aid physical, mental, and emotional renewal, also decision-making. On the physical level Bloodstone strengthens the kidneys, liver, and spleen, thereby promoting detoxification.

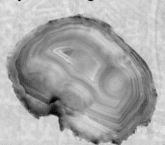

Agate

The Fire agate or the brown/brown-black Moss agate are best choices for the Root Chakra. Use them if your chakra is deficient in energy, to enhance self-esteem, assist physical and emotional security, and help you take a more balanced perspective on life - particularly through eliminating negativity.

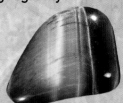

Smoky Quartz

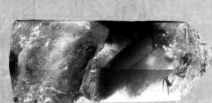

A form of quartz ranging from light to dark grey and black. Another excellent "grounding" crystal that encourages you to focus on the present moment. It is said to activate survival instincts and improve intuition about challenges and problems. A useful stone for dissolving negative energies and emotional blockages.

Tiger's Eye

A silicon dioxide with an iridescent cat's eye effect. Colours range from black to dark brown, with fibrous yellow or golden brown inclusions. Used at the Root Chakra this crystal focuses energy needed to meet challenges and encourages optimism and discipline. It also helps shed light on the practical steps needed to achieve goals.

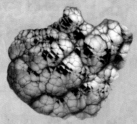

Hematite

Colours range from brown-red to dark grey or black, all with a metallic sheen. This is an excellent "grounding" crystal that also assists in shifting mental limitations holding you back from trying new directions by dissolving negativity associated with fear of new ventures.

PETER (see also pp.40-1)

This layout was used for Peter. All five crystals were placed over his Root Chakra to help him overcome challenges he faced after his mother's death:

▽ **Moss agate** - to build up low self-esteem, giving emotional and physical security;

▽ **Bloodstone** - to boost the renewal process and help clear physical blockages;

▽ **Hematite** - to help focus on the potential for a fulfilling social and work life and assist in dissolving negativity;

▽ **Tiger's eye** - to encourage the optimism and discipline needed to move forward and become secure and independent;

▽ **Smoky quartz** - to help Peter face future challenges with enthusiasm.

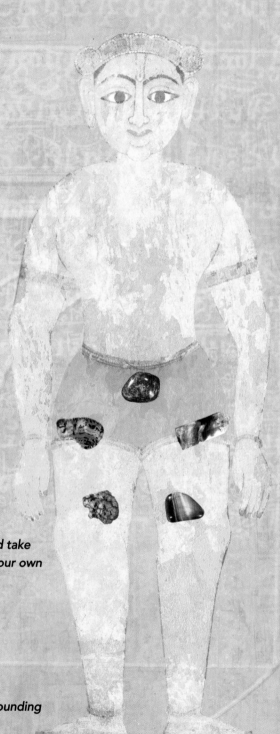

Approach crystal healing with an open mind and take the time to choose and position crystals, with your own needs and wishes uppermost.

▽ *Choose a warm, comfortable place.*

▽ *Ensure you are not going to be disturbed.*

▽ *Play gentle music or nature sounds.*

▽ *Burn incense or scented candles.*

▽ *Wear loose clothes.*

▽ *Go to the bathroom first.*

▽ *Have a glass of water for rehydration and grounding afterwards.*

▽ *Cleanse and tune the crystals (see p.27).*

MEDITATION: ROOT CHAKRA

Before you start
Choose a leisurely and relaxed time to meditate.
▽ Sit or lie before your altar (see pp.40-1). Let the colours, symbols, and associ-ations inspire you.
▽ Create atmosphere with oils, candles, or incense.
▽ Tape the words if you like. Dots indicate a pause.

1. Breathe slowly and deeply through your nose.

2. Tense each set of muscles in turn, from feet to head ... then relax them, gradually sinking into the floor or chair ...

3. Visualize yourself in perfect surroundings. You are safe, warm, and secure.

4. Who are the people in this happy place with you? Acknowledge each one ... Feel their love radiate as a reddish golden glow penetrating every cell of your being, filling you with joy ...

5. Imagine your inner mother looking benevolently down on you. Sense her smile enveloping you like a soft cloak ... Know that she will never let you down. She is part of you and will always protect you.

6. Approach your inner mother. Hug, kiss, or link arms. Enjoy the sensation ... Take time to get to know one another. Enjoy the sensation of re-acquaintance and trust ...

7. Let her give you a present. Examine it. Feel it, smell it, admire the colour and shape. If appropriate, taste it ...
Thank your mother and tell her you will treasure her gift. It is yours to keep and recall every time you feel abandoned or victimized.

8. As you hold your gift, feel the energy of your inner mother's love channelled into your Root Chakra ... Imagine this chakra as a four-petalled lotus rotating like a wheel ...

9. Focus on the smooth motion of the chakra and the warm, red glow that fills that part of your body, flow-ing down your legs to connect you with the Earth ...

10. Enjoy the reassuring sensation of groundedness, security, and stability before bringing your attention back to your everyday surroundings.

DAILY QUESTIONS

▽ Does your home reflect who you truly are? If not, how can you change it?

▽ What reward have you given yourself today? A gift, an affirmation, praise, or good turn?

▽ Have you focused on abundance or lack today? List things representing abundance (family support/money saved).

▽ How could you improve financial security? List weekly expenses. Where could savings be made?

▽ Have you lost contact with family or friends? How could you re-establish links? (Make approaches through love, not obligation.)

▽ How do you honour your body? Do you address diet, exercise, and relaxation regularly?

AFFIRMATIONS

▽ My body is becoming more important to me. I nurture it constantly.

▽ I am taking responsibility for my life. I can cope with any situation.

▽ I recognize the abundance of love, trust, and care surrounding me.

▽ My internal mother is always here for me, protecting, nourishing, and soothing me.

▽ I deserve the best that life has to offer. My needs are always met.

▽ I am connected to Mother Earth and know the security of being grounded in reality, in the moment.

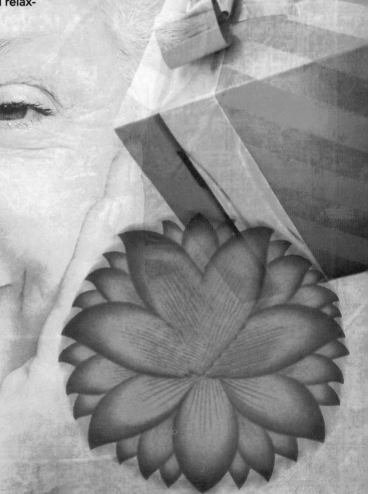

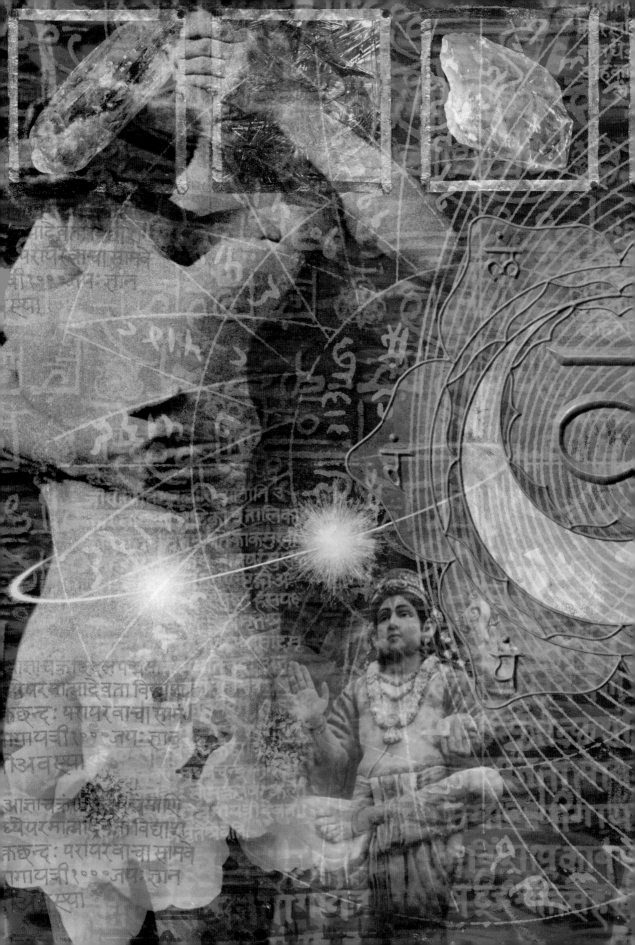

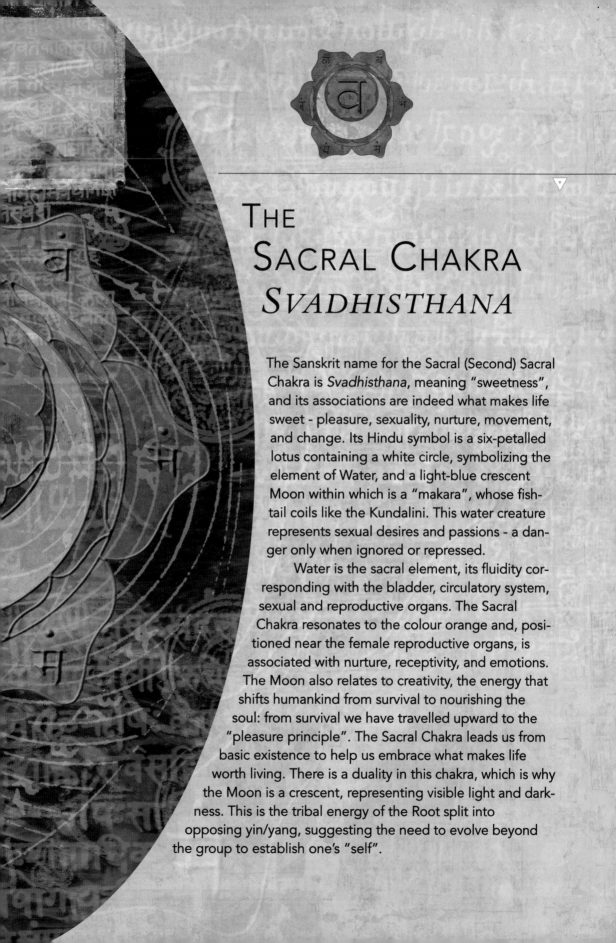

THE
SACRAL CHAKRA
SVADHISTHANA

The Sanskrit name for the Sacral (Second) Sacral Chakra is *Svadhisthana*, meaning "sweetness", and its associations are indeed what makes life sweet - pleasure, sexuality, nurture, movement, and change. Its Hindu symbol is a six-petalled lotus containing a white circle, symbolizing the element of Water, and a light-blue crescent Moon within which is a "makara", whose fish-tail coils like the Kundalini. This water creature represents sexual desires and passions - a danger only when ignored or repressed.

Water is the sacral element, its fluidity corresponding with the bladder, circulatory system, sexual and reproductive organs. The Sacral Chakra resonates to the colour orange and, positioned near the female reproductive organs, is associated with nurture, receptivity, and emotions. The Moon also relates to creativity, the energy that shifts humankind from survival to nourishing the soul: from survival we have travelled upward to the "pleasure principle". The Sacral Chakra leads us from basic existence to help us embrace what makes life worth living. There is a duality in this chakra, which is why the Moon is a crescent, representing visible light and darkness. This is the tribal energy of the Root split into opposing yin/yang, suggesting the need to evolve beyond the group to establish one's "self".

Sacral Chakra Correspondences

This chart for the Sacral (Second) Chakra provides a "ready reference" of inspirations to use when you carry out practical exercises such as assembling your altar arrangements (see pp.54-5) or choosing appropriate stones for crystal work (see pp.58-9). It will also help you with the various images you will need when composing your own meditations and visualizations. Incorporate as many of these symbols and themes as are appropriate to your needs.

By re-acquainting yourself regularly with this chakra chart as a prelude to the section on the Sacral Chakra, you will help to keep your mind focused on related issues. This includes an acceptance of the desire to enjoy a pleasurable lifestyle and to embrace whatever change is necessary to bring that about.

To make your Sacral Chakra work successful and enjoyable you should prepare yourself by attending to certain practical requirements (see pp.25 and 59). Finding pleasure in life's activities generates the enthusiasm and energy to take on even more creative projects, whether concerning family, business, relationships, or social activities. This is what the Sacral Chakra can bring you.

CHAKRA CHARACTERISTICS

See which of the following characteristics of excessive ("too open"), deficient ("blocked"), and balanced chakra energy you can related to - and then determine (should you choose) to take the necessary action, using the tools and techniques outlined in this chapter.

Too open (chakra spins too fast) - emotionally unbalanced, a fantasist, manipulative, sexually addictive
Blocked (chakra spins sluggishly or not at all) - over-sensitive, hard on him/herself, feels guilty for no reason, frigid or impotent
Balanced (chakra maintains equilibrium and spins at correct vibrational speed) - trusting, expressive, attuned to his/her own feelings, creative

THE SACRAL CHAKRA

Sanskrit Name
Svadhisthana

Meaning
Sweetness

Location
Lower abdomen,
between navel
& genitals

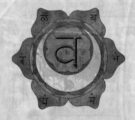

Symbol
Six orange-red petals
containing a second lotus
flower and a crescent
moon. Within the moon
lies the "makara", a fish-
tailed alligator with
coiled tail.

Associated Colour
Orange

Element
Water

Ruling Planet
Pluto

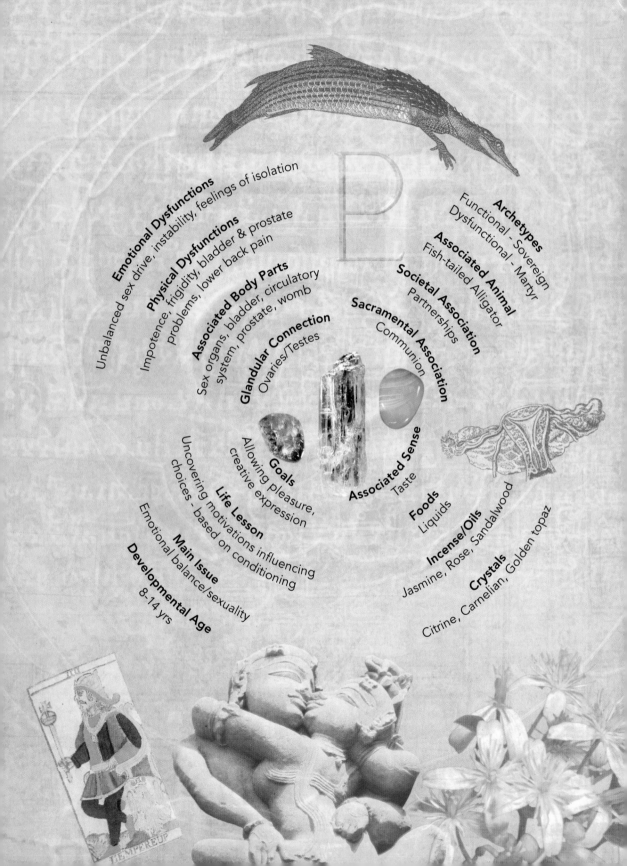

Emotional Dysfunctions
Unbalanced sex drive, instability, feelings of isolation

Physical Dysfunctions
Impotence, frigidity, bladder & prostate problems, lower back pain

Associated Body Parts
Sex organs, bladder, circulatory system, prostate, womb

Glandular Connection
Ovaries/Testes

Goals
Allowing pleasure, creative expression

Life Lesson
Uncovering motivations influencing choices - based on conditioning

Main Issue
Emotional balance/sexuality

Developmental Age
8-14 yrs

Archetypes
Functional - Sovereign
Dysfunctional - Martyr

Associated Animal
Fish-tailed Alligator

Societal Association
Partnerships

Sacramental Association
Communion

Associated Sense
Taste

Foods
Liquids

Incense/Oils
Jasmine, Rose, Sandalwood

Crystals
Citrine, Carnelian, Golden topaz

ARCHETYPES: SACRAL CHAKRA

The Sacral (Second) Chakra further develops the themes of
the Root (First) Chakra of personal responsibility and self-
expression. Its archetypes are the Sovereign and the Martyr,
which are involved with our attitudes concerning abundance
and how much we believe that we deserve to enjoy life.
These two associations represent the polarities of pleasure
and fulfilment, and suffering and sacrifice.

Martyrs are less likely than Victims to blame external influences for what they perceive as a life of suffering, but share
a similar belief that they don't deserve anything better.
Martyrdom involves being entrenched in a pit of self-pity
with no motivation to shift the negative attitudes contributing to the situation. Martyrs' lives are steeped in a sense of
lack, which underpins a justification for not changing beliefs
and behaviours because there is just not enough good fortune in the world to go round - and they have drawn the
short straw. So they whine and complain, but never take any
action. Theirs is a passive acceptance of life rather than the
active desire to change and develop. Without a proper
regard for personal needs and desires, mothers very often
develop into Martyrs.

The positive side of this coin is the Sovereign - the archetype of those who allow the good things of life to be part of
their everyday experiences. They are magnetic personalities
whom everyone enjoys being with, in contrast with guilt-
inducing Martyrs. These individuals do not necessarily live
charmed lives, it's simply that when confronted with a challenging situation they see the positive opportunities for
growth and development. They are content to take the
rough with the smooth in the knowledge that life is all about
shades of light and dark, positives and negatives, good and
bad. They know that winter always turns into spring. Their
more developed inner world gives them permission to
rejoice in their own achievements. Nurturing their own
desires is a high priority for the Sovereigns of this world. To
them life is bountiful and they, as much as anyone else,
deserve a share in the beauty and rewards that surround
them, including sexual fulfilment. Sex to them is something
to be celebrated and enjoyed rather than being a sinful

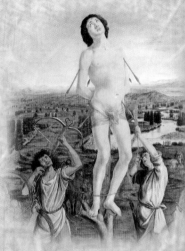

DESERVED UNHAPPINESS

The mental self-flagella-
tion of Martyrs comes
from the belief that they
deserve all the unhappi-
ness and misery that
comes their way. Many
Western societies and
religious groups encour-
age this belief through
messages such as; "Life
is tough", "You only get
what you want through
hard work and sacrifice"
and "Think of others
rather than yourself".

activity; a view that many Western cultures seem to espouse. Taking a creative approach to their sexuality, Sovereigns achieve fulfilment in this important area of their lives.

Because they are always on the look-out for the benefits rather than disadvantages, they tend to find that that's exactly what life offers to them.

THE SOVEREIGN

These individuals are not necessarily any luckier than anyone else, but when present- ed with a landscape they will home in on the flowers, the blades of grass, and the butterflies rather than the litter, the dog mess, and the ants.

THE MARTYR

Martyrs revel in self-pity - they are the "poor me's" of society. They make what they regard as sacrifices for others that are rarely appreciated or even acknowledged.

By undertaking the meditation, daily questions, and affirmations on pages 60-1 you will be able to explore the theme of passion in all areas of your life and shift the shackles of martyrdom which may be repressing you.

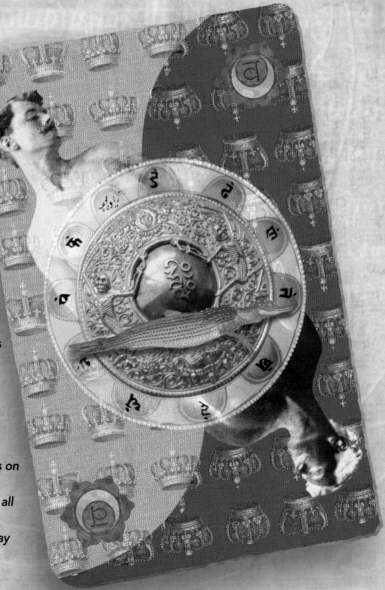

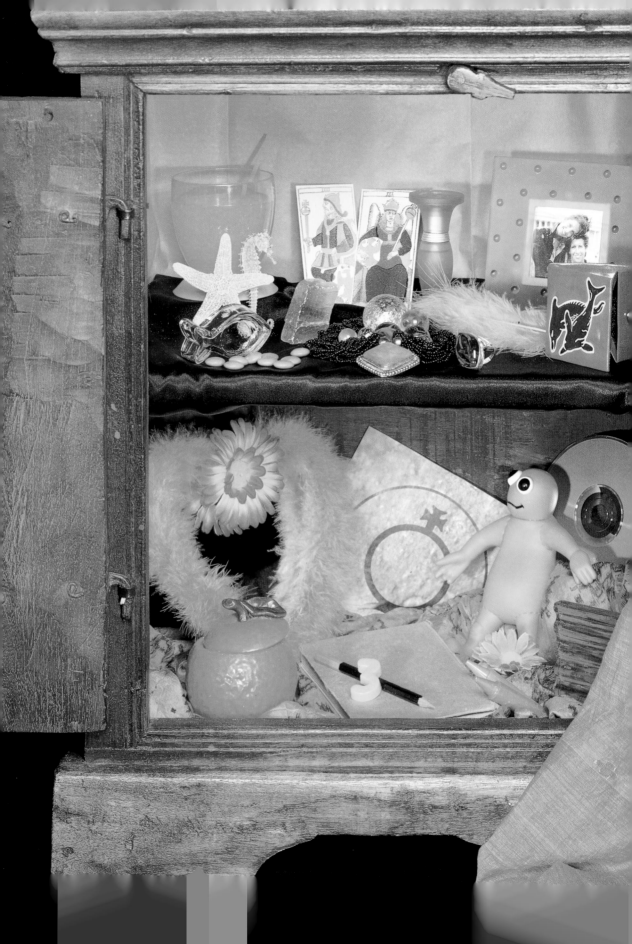

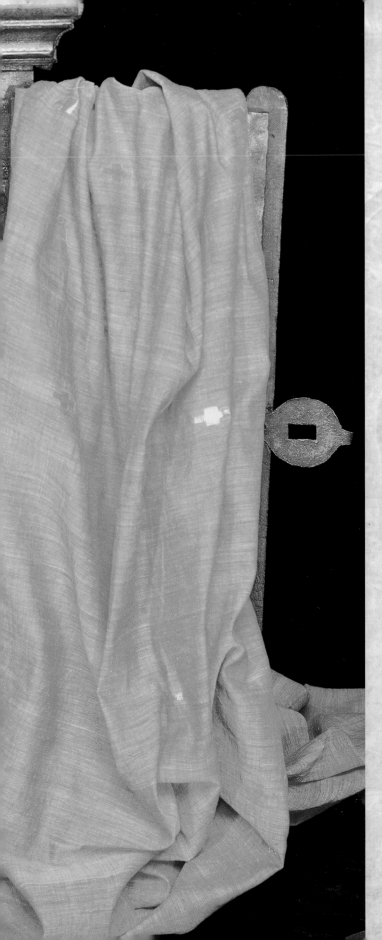

ALTAR:
SACRAL CHAKRA

Barbara created this altar in order to help stabilize and strengthen a dysfunctional Sacral Chakra, after her relationship with Mark had reached rock bottom. Barbara was feeling increasingly isolated, despite having been with Mark for six years. Haunted by the memory of her philandering father, Barbara was constantly looking for signs that Mark was being unfaithful - which he denied. Emotional see-sawing was having a detrimental impact on their sex life and this, in turn, was affecting her work. Having being inspired to take action to change her negativity and self-pity by a supportive friend, Barbara incorporated the following items:

▽ Orange-shaped candle, for sweetness in relationships
▽ Heart-shaped mirror to reflect back love to the Self
▽ Orange-covered personal note-book containing love poems
▽ Barbara's lucky number - three
▽ A childhood toy, as a reminder of pleasure and fun
▽ A record of love songs
▽ Dolphins, an orange starfish and a seahorse - all water symbols, the key Sacral element
▽ A photo of Barbara and Mark
▽ An Amber ring, orange stone necklace, and a golden Topaz
▽ Sovereign and Martyr archetypes
▽ Orange feathers for sensuality
▽ Jasmine perfume
▽ Orange silk brought back from a happy holiday with Mark

This altar is Barbara's attempt to work on the Sacral Chakra. It is a case study, for inspiration. Choose objects of personal significance.

EXERCISES: SACRAL CHAKRA

Try not to be inhibited when trying out these exercises, both of which are designed to stimulate the Sacral Chakra. If you think you may feel uncomfortable or vulnerable doing the Pelvic Rock Exercise (facing page), in particular, ensure that you are somewhere private, make a determined mental effort to enjoy yourself - and think of Elvis Presley or Michael Jackson!

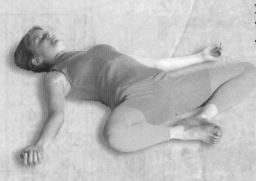

1. Lie on your back with your arms at 45-degree angles to your body. Bend your knees and pull your feet up toward your genital area as far as feels comfortable. Allow your knees to fall out to the sides, stretching the insides of your thighs.

2. Don't worry if your knees don't touch the floor; much will depend on your age and flexibility. Just maintain this open feeling and be comfortable with it, without forcing your body to do anything it doesn't want to do.

3. Bring your knees together and up toward your chest. Enclose your knees with clasped hands and allow the weight of your arms to press your legs inward.

4. Focus first on your lower back and try gently pressing yourself downward into the floor. Then shift focus to your pelvis and press your tailbone into the floor so that, as you change from one focus to the other, you engage in a gentle rocking movement. Imagine a warm orange liquid swishing inside you, so that every part of your sacral area is massaged inwardly.

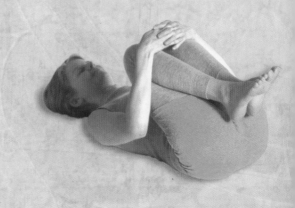

PELVIC ROCK EXERCISE

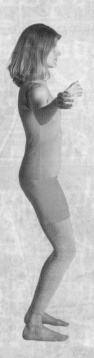

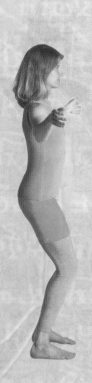

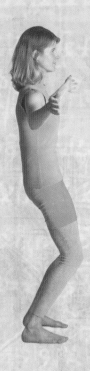

1. Stand with your feet a shoulder-width apart, knees slightly bent, and your arms extended as far as is comfortable, and to keep you balanced.

2. Tilt your pelvis - the area between your hips and lower abdomen - backward while keeping the rest of your body static.

3. Thrust your pelvis forward in a swinging motion. Once you have got the hang of this exercise, you should be able to rock your pelvis rhythmically in a continuous motion while focusing your mind on the smooth spinning of an orange disk at the Sacral Chakra.

KEY CRYSTALS: SACRAL CHAKRA

The goals of emotional stability, creative expression, and experiencing pleasure in life, which relate to this chakra, are enhanced by the crystals suggested here. The association with the colour range is a loose one. Suggestions vary from the pale, silvery sheen of Moonstone to the golden and amber hues of Topaz, Citrine, and Carnelian. (See also pp.26-7 for information on Crystal Healing.)

CITRINE

A pale yellow-brown or amber-coloured member of the Quartz family that encourages the openness needed to tackle emotional stagnancy in relationships. Citrine helps support and develop emotional maturity, particularly for those who are experiencing periods of instability in their emotional life.

CARNELIAN

A red-orange Chalcedony that helps stimulate initiative and dispel apathy and passivity. It is particularly useful for promoting the physical energy needed to take action in emotionally challenging circumstances. Carnelian is also said to help dissipate sorrow from the emotional self.

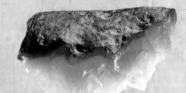

MOONSTONE

This milky-sheened member of the feldspar group is usually colourless, white, or silver. It helps enhance your feminine side. Benefits include a calming of the emotions so that you can take a more objective view of a situation, and balance oversensitivity. It is also said to arouse a greater feeling of tenderness and compassion toward yourself.

RUTILATED QUARTZ

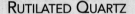

Quartz crystals are invaluable tools to use on any of the chakras. This form contains needle-like crystals of Rutile, giving the stone its unique appearance. As such it combines the benefits of Quartz for meditation, spiritual development, and healing, with those of Rutile - a crystal said to help stabilize relationships and emotional imbalances.

GOLDEN TOPAZ

A valuable crystal for actively stimulating the first three chakras. Used on the Sacral Chakra Golden topaz helps promote inner peace and lightness of spirit, in turn helping you take a new perspective on problems. It is also thought of as a "battery" that helps energize those physically, mentally, or emotionally under the weather.

BARBARA (see also pp.54-5)

This layout was used on Barbara, who agreed with her healer to tackle deeper problems concerning lack of emotional maturity before moving on to deal with issues connected with her partner. Hence her layout consisted of a design over the Sacral area using tumblestones of Citrine only. First of all, Barbara was encouraged to hold her hand over the crystals, with eyes closed, and to sense any "pull" drawing her to particular stones. These are signs that the vibration of those crystals matched Barbara's own bodily resonance. She was encouraged to visualize a warm, orange liquid washing through her Sacral area, dissolving fears about male infidelity and helping to recognize that past experiences do not necessarily have an impact on the present - unless you allow them to.

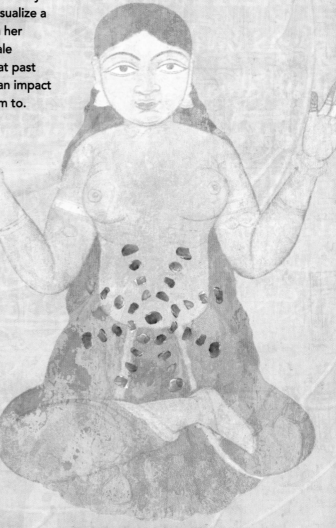

Approach crystal healing with an open mind and take the time to choose and position crystals with your own needs and wishes uppermost.

▽ *Choose a warm, comfortable place.*
▽ *Ensure you are not going to be disturbed.*
▽ *Play gentle music or nature sounds.*
▽ *Burn incense or scented candles.*
▽ *Wear loose clothes.*
▽ *Go to the bathroom first.*
▽ *Have a glass of water to rehydrate and ground you afterwards.*
▽ *Cleanse and tune the crystals (see p.27).*

MEDITATION: SACRAL CHAKRA

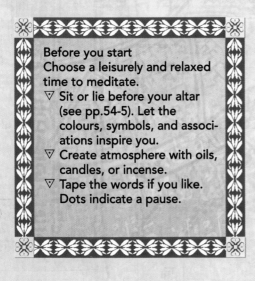

Before you start
Choose a leisurely and relaxed
time to meditate.
▽ Sit or lie before your altar
   (see pp.54-5). Let the
   colours, symbols, and associations inspire you.
▽ Create atmosphere with oils,
   candles, or incense.
▽ Tape the words if you like.
   Dots indicate a pause.

*1. As you lie motionless, become aware of change and
movement that continues in your body ...
your heartbeat ... blood flow around your body ...
cellular activity that invisibly rejuvenates your whole
being. Your every breath celebrates life ...
nourishing you with everything you
need for a healthy, enjoyable life.*

*2. Focus on the gentle movement of your abdomen as you breathe.
Imagine it filled with a warm, orange glow, representing joy and
vitality, both of which are available to you in abundance ...*

*3. Bring to mind a pleasurable experience ...
Recollect all the senses that will bring that
moment back to life for you now ...
Remember how you felt ...
 the colours around you ...
textures ... shapes ... sounds ... smells ... tastes.*

*4. Shift that image to your abdomen so that the warm, orange
glow suffuses it, magnifying the experience and making it even
more satisfying and joyous ...
Surrender your body to the pleasures of that moment ...
something you deserve to experience every day of your life,
and can have again every time you put your mind to it ...*

*5. Know that your life can be a succession of wonderful, beneficial
experiences if you choose it to be so ...
Determine to look for the opportunities, the love, the joy, and the
fun in all you do today. You deserve it.*

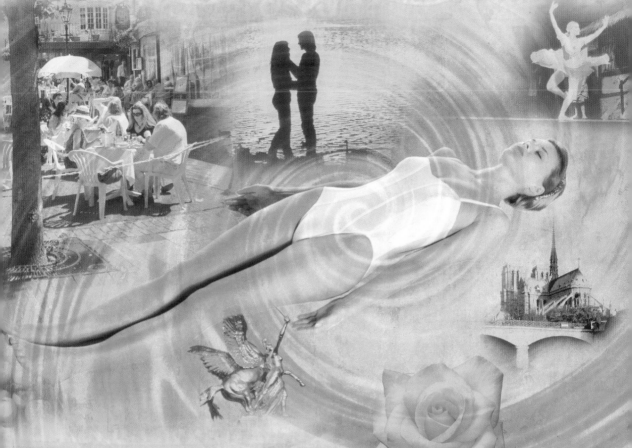

DAILY QUESTIONS

▽ How much are you prepared to embrace change? Change one small thing today.

▽ How creative are you sexually? Discuss your fantasies with your partner.

▽ What sacrifices do you make to suit others? Dysfunctional relationships are toxic to both. Try saying "no" next time. Don't explain.

▽ Do you respect your female and male sides? It is alright to be soft one day, assertive the next. Different situations require different responses.

▽ Is it better to give than to receive? Accepting gifts, with pleasure, gives others something back. Do you deny them the joy of giving?

▽ Do you believe that for your desires to be met you first have to make a sacrifice? Focus on someone for whom life is sweet. Try mirroring them. Have you made a shift in your beliefs?

AFFIRMATIONS

▽ I am moving toward a time when I am totally happy and fulfilled. Life offers me everything I need for that journey.

▽ I am worthy of love and sexual pleasure.

▽ I have a right to express my desires to myself and others.

▽ Who I am is good enough.

▽ Life is unfolding as it should.

▽ I am prepared to honour my body and feel good about my sexuality.

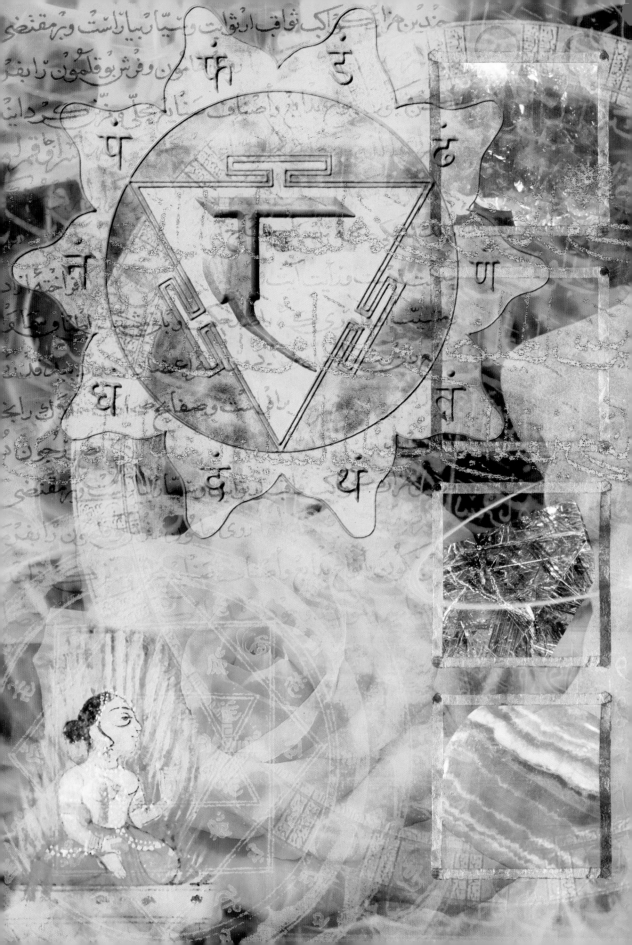

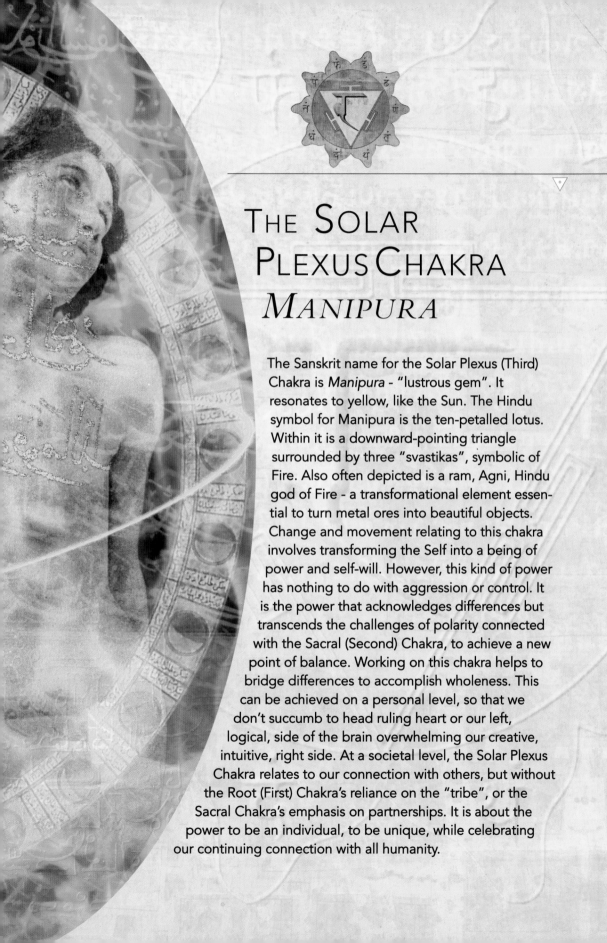

THE SOLAR PLEXUS CHAKRA

MANIPURA

The Sanskrit name for the Solar Plexus (Third) Chakra is *Manipura* - "lustrous gem". It resonates to yellow, like the Sun. The Hindu symbol for Manipura is the ten-petalled lotus. Within it is a downward-pointing triangle surrounded by three "svastikas", symbolic of Fire. Also often depicted is a ram, Agni, Hindu god of Fire - a transformational element essential to turn metal ores into beautiful objects. Change and movement relating to this chakra involves transforming the Self into a being of power and self-will. However, this kind of power has nothing to do with aggression or control. It is the power that acknowledges differences but transcends the challenges of polarity connected with the Sacral (Second) Chakra, to achieve a new point of balance. Working on this chakra helps to bridge differences to accomplish wholeness. This can be achieved on a personal level, so that we don't succumb to head ruling heart or our left, logical, side of the brain overwhelming our creative, intuitive, right side. At a societal level, the Solar Plexus Chakra relates to our connection with others, but without the Root (First) Chakra's reliance on the "tribe", or the Sacral Chakra's emphasis on partnerships. It is about the power to be an individual, to be unique, while celebrating our continuing connection with all humanity.

SOLAR PLEXUS CHAKRA CORRESPONDENCES

This chart for the Solar Plexus (Third) Chakra identifies the associations and symbolisms linked with this particular chakra. As such it provides a "ready reference" of inspirations to use when carrying out practical exercises such as assembling your altar (see pp.68-9) or choosing appropriate stones for crystal work (see pp.72-3). This chart will also help you with the various images you will need when composing your own meditations and visualizations. Incorporate as many of these symbols and themes as you feel is appropriate to your needs.

By re-acquainting yourself regularly with this chakra chart as a prelude to the entire section on the Solar Plexus Chakra, you will help focus your mind on its related issues. These include the development of your self-esteem as a precursor to achieving true personal power.

To make your chakra journey successful and enjoyable you should prepare yourself by attending to certain preliminaries (see pp.25 and 73). By strengthening and stimulating the Solar Plexus Chakra you will reach a state in which you can shake off the fears of rejection, criticism, and standing apart from the group and create your own, unique, identity. One that is founded on self-acceptance, self-respect, and the ability to take risks in the knowledge that you can handle any situation with which you are faced. This is true inner, personal power.

CHAKRA CHARACTERISTICS

See which of the following characteristics of excessive ("too open"), deficient ("blocked"), and balanced chakra energy you can relate to - and then determine (should you choose) to take the necessary action, using the tools and techniques outlined in this chapter.

Too open (chakra spins too fast) - angry, controlling, workaholic, judgemental and superior
Blocked (chakra spins sluggishly or not at all) - overly concerned with what others think, fearful of being alone, insecure, needs constant reassurance
Balanced (chakra maintains equilibrium and spins at correct vibrational speed) - respects self and others, has personal power, spontaneous, uninhibited

THE SOLAR PLEXUS CHAKRA

Sanskrit Name
Manipura

Meaning
Lustrous gem

Location
Between navel & base of sternum

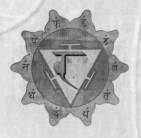

Symbol
A ten-petalled lotus flower containing a downward-pointing triangle surrounded by three T-shaped svastikas, or Hindu symbols of fire.

Associated Colour
Yellow

Element
Fire

Ruling Planets
Mars, Sun

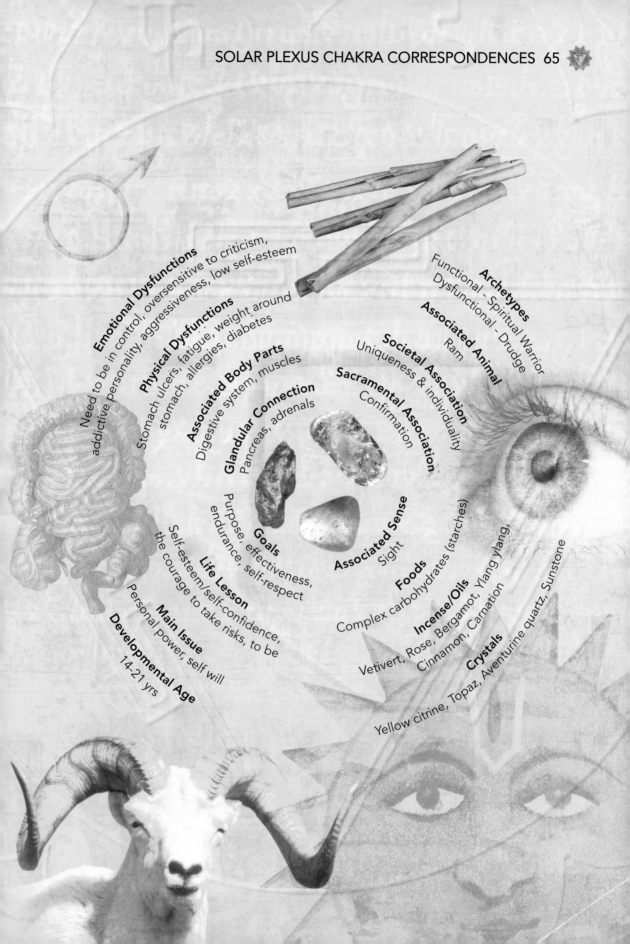

Emotional Dysfunctions
Need to be in control, oversensitive to criticism, addictive personality, aggressiveness, low self-esteem

Physical Dysfunctions
Stomach ulcers, fatigue, weight around stomach, allergies, diabetes

Associated Body Parts
Digestive system, muscles

Glandular Connection
Pancreas, adrenals

Goals
Purpose, effectiveness, endurance, self-respect

Life Lesson
Self-esteem/self-confidence, the courage to take risks, to be

Main Issue
Personal power, self will

Developmental Age
14-21 yrs

Archetypes
Functional - Spiritual Warrior
Dysfunctional - Drudge

Associated Animal
Ram

Societal Association
Uniqueness & individuality

Sacramental Association
Confirmation

Associated Sense
Sight

Foods
Complex carbohydrates (starches)

Incense/Oils
Vetivert, Rose, Bergamot, Ylang ylang, Cinnamon, Carnation

Crystals
Yellow citrine, Topaz, Aventurine quartz, Sunstone

Archetypes: Solar Plexus Chakra

While the first two chakras have been concerned with our external relationships - the Root (First) Chakra with the group mind and the Sacral (Second) with specific relationships - the Solar Plexus (Third) Chakra is more internally focused: to our relationship with ourselves. The ways in which we demonstrate our self-esteem and personal power is played out in the archetypes associated with this chakra - the Drudge and Spiritual Warrior.

The Drudge is not as dysfunctional as the Victim and Martyr of the first two chakras, but continues the themes of lack of acknowledgement and reward. Drudges hand over the responsibility for their happiness by their submissiveness and dependence on others. They commonly regard being loveable only in terms of what they do, not who they are. So they unconsciously look for relationships that reinforce that view. Hence the Drudge archetype can become involved with bullying, dominant partners (who are often violent and abusive) or work colleagues whose self-importance is fuelled by the self-effacing, easily manipulated, Drudge. Unfortunately the outside approval that Drudges desperately seek is not forthcoming, because this only happens when we learn to honour and value ourselves. Their inner chant of "I am not worthy" needs to be erased in order for a true sense of self-worth to find its voice.

In direct contrast, the Spiritual Warrior archetype is the hero or heroine who operates instinctively in their interactions with others, and always from a position of equality. The Solar Plexus Chakra is associated with the digestive system. When we ignore, reject, or suppress our psychic sensitivity this can lead to blockages in this area, resulting in excess weight around the middle, digestive problems, and stomach ulcers.

By meeting constant rejection or conflict, the Spiritual Warriors of myth and legend were forced to look inside themselves to make sense of those sets of circumstances and give them meaning. It is a truly powerful archetype when a spiritual philosophy of growth and development through facing life's obstacles is combined with acting with integrity, no matter how unpopular or inexplicable to others

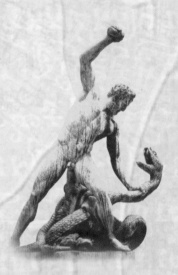

Myths and Legends

The fairy story of Cinderella and her relationship with her two ugly half-sisters is an example of the Drudge mentality in operation. In stories the Spiritual Warrior is the pauper who confronts a king, or the knight who faces the power of wizards. In mythology the Labours of Hercules is a prime example. In such stories, logic and reason are acted out in conjunction with the "psychic" abilities known as "hunches" or "gut" feelings.

those actions may be. The attributes of this functional archetype are the precursors to the power of love that is connected with the next chakra on our journey - the Heart. Because only by truly loving and honouring ourselves can we hope to act out of love and compassion toward others.

THE SPIRITUAL WARRIOR

The power of the Spiritual Warrior lies in inner strength, tempered by a belief that guidance comes from a Divine force. This strength becomes honed and refined through facing and overcoming external challenges.

THE DRUDGE

A drudge mentality depends on others for recognition and approval, investing everyone else with qualities and power that they wished they owned themselves (and, indeed, do own - if only they could acknowledge that).

Meditation, daily questions, and affirmations (pp.74-5) continue these themes, to help you to throw off subservient Drudge tendencies and take on the inner strength of the Spiritual Warrior.

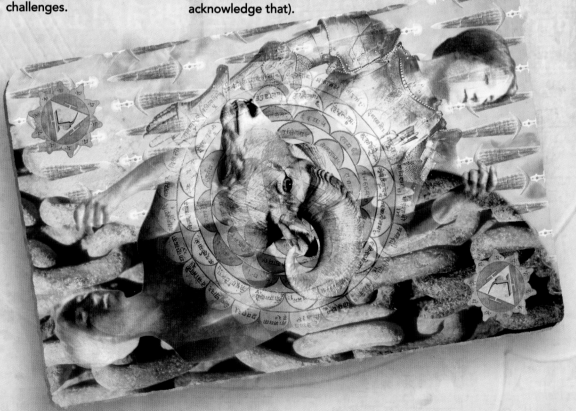

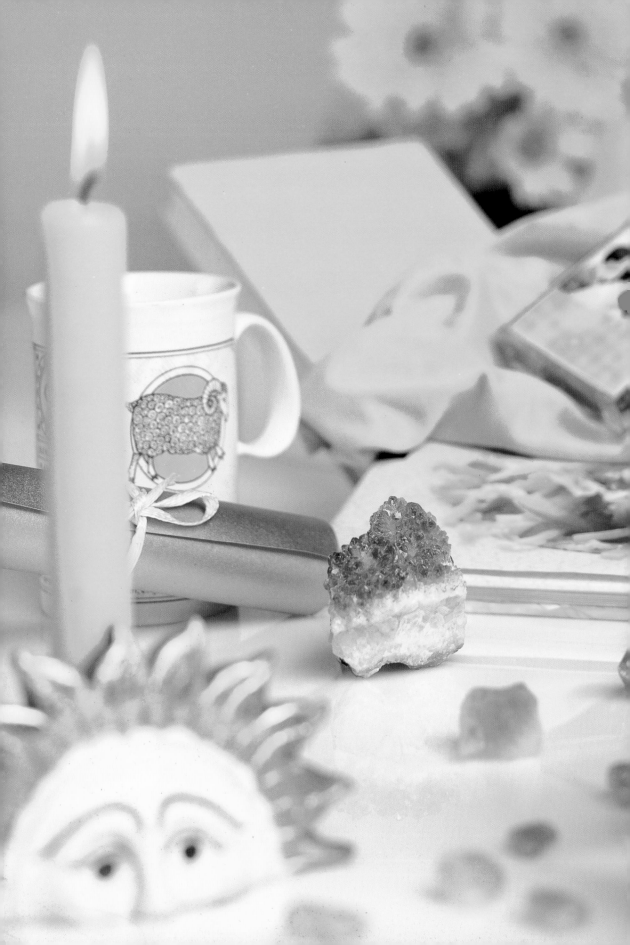

ALTAR:
SOLAR PLEXUS CHAKRA

Gina didn't like the workaholic she'd become and was determined to relinquish her need to control everything. She realized that she had "shut off" areas of her life because of work. Things came to a head when she was turned down for promotion because of poor teamwork. Gina recognized that her fear of delegating was fuelled by a need to dominate. Her quest for power was based on underlying lack of confidence and she had constructed an abrasive attitude in order to cope. Her personal life was non-existent because of long hours at work. She felt constantly exhausted and had recurring irritable bowel syndrome. Fired up by a new sense of purpose, Gina collected the following items:

▽ Golden yellow cloth bought on a recent business trip
▽ Mug with Aries, the ram
▽ Self-help book for addictives
▽ Audio tape programme to help her develop team skills
▽ Her goals and objectives for the year ahead, on gold paper
▽ Cookery book with inspiring, easy recipes for single people
▽ Golden "Sun" candle holder with yellow candle
▽ Large chunk of Citrine for focusing on in self-esteem meditations
▽ Bowl containing goldfish in her Feng Shui career location

This altar is Gina's attempt to work on the Solar Plexus Chakra. It is a case study, for inspiration. Choose objects which have personal significance for you.

EXERCISE: SOLAR PLEXUS CHAKRA

In this free-flowing visualization walk, your body "follows" your Solar Plexus, so select an area that is big enough for you to move around with ease and in which you won't be distracted or interrupted. Wear loose, comfortable clothing in a temperate environment so that you will not become too hot. Play gentle background music if this won't distract you from the visualizations. It might help to close your eyes, but make sure there are no objects that you could bump into.

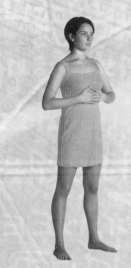

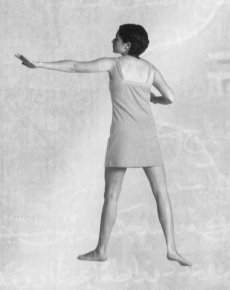

1. Stand with your feet a shoulder-width apart and your hands placed on your Solar Plexus. Visualize a golden yellow sphere vibrating under your palms, pulsating with light and energy. Sense this yellow glow extending out from your Solar Plexus Chakra to the rest of your body. Become aware of the power that is now available to you, from the top of your head to the tips of your toes.

2. Still keeping this vision in your mind's eye, allow your Solar Plexus to direct the movement of your body as if it were a ball of light trying to escape from your stomach area. Let it spontaneously guide your movements around the room for a few minutes. Keeping your spine straight, allow your arms to swing out to the sides and twist your body to follow their motion. Continue with this motion as you intuitively follow the direction in which your Solar Plexus wants you to go.

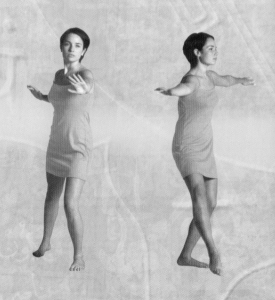

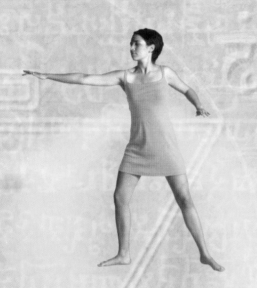

3. Acknowledge any inhibited thoughts that enter your head, but let them pass by, like clouds on a summer's day. Try not to concentrate on anything other than the gentle, flowing movements of your body and arms. Take this opportunity to drift off into your own world for as long as you feel comfortable, all the time keeping your mind focused on the powerful ball of light emanating from your stomach area.

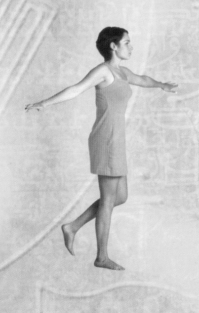

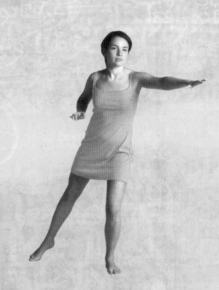

Allow yourself to become abandoned to the power within you, shutting off the inner voice of "shouldn'ts" and "can'ts".

KEY CRYSTALS: SOLAR PLEXUS CHAKRA

The metaphor of the sun as related to the Solar Plexus core theme of power corresponds with the yellow hues of Third Chakra crystals. Your specific choice will be determined by whether the dysfunction you wish to overcome is physical, mental, or emotional. (See also pp.26-7 for information on Crystal Healing.)

YELLOW CITRINE
When used on the Solar Plexus this crystal helps individuals access their personal power. It enhances self-confidence and can help overcome an attraction to addictive substances, which is a common dysfunction of this chakra. On a physical level Yellow citrine is of great benefit for digestive problems.

CALCITE
This crystal comes in many colours and shapes, but the golden or yellow forms are most suitable for the Solar Plexus. Calcite is said to intensify the energy of this chakra, helping to "kick-start" it after removing blockages. It is also excellent for problems associated with the dysfunction of the pancreas, kidneys, and spleen.

SUNSTONE
Despite its name, Sunstone comes in a range of colours as well as yellow and orange. Its speckling reflections are due to inclusions of Hematite and Goethite. In Ancient Greece it represented the Sun God, bringing good fortune to anyone who wore it. It is useful for reducing tension in the stomach and for relief of ulcers.

MALACHITE
A green crystal with characteristic banding, it helps to link the Solar Plexus to the Heart (on which it can also be placed) to promote the compassion needed to ensure that personal power doesn't become misplaced. This stone is particularly good for helping to remember dreams and is excellent for meditation.

GINA (see also pp.68-9)

This layout was used for Gina. She chose a combination of Malachite, Yellow citrine, and Calcite. In addition she achieved a total energy boost to combat exhaustion by using nine single-terminated Clear quartz crystals:

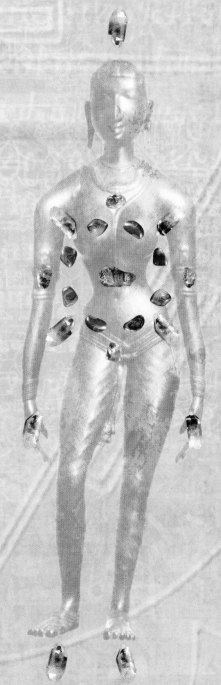

▽ **Quartz** - in each hand, pointed end toward the shoulders; one toward the sole of each foot; one pointing at the Crown. The other four, with pointed ends toward the Solar Plexus, surrounded the coloured crystals over the chakra;

▽ **Yellow citrine** - to unblock stagnant energy causing irritable bowel syndrome and to boost self-confidence;

▽ **Calcite** - in combination with the Clear quartz gave a much-needed energy boost;

▽ **Malachite** - helped Gina direct personal power in a more balanced, compassionate, way to benefit her colleagues.

Approach crystal healing with an open mind and take the time to choose and position crystals with your needs and wishes upper-most.

▽ *Choose a warm, comfortable place.*
▽ *Ensure you are not going to be disturbed.*
▽ *Play gentle music or nature sounds.*
▽ *Burn incense or scented candles.*
▽ *Wear loose clothes.*
▽ *Go to the bathroom first.*
▽ *Have a glass of water to rehydrate and ground you afterwards.*
▽ *Cleanse and tune the crystals (see p.27).*

MEDITATION: SOLAR PLEXUS CHAKRA

Before you start
Choose a leisurely and relaxed time to meditate.
▽ Sit or lie before your altar (see pp.68-9). Let the colours, symbols, and associations inspire you.
▽ Create atmosphere with oils, candles, or incense.
▽ Tape the words if you like. Dots indicate a pause.

1. You are on a path that winds up into the distance.
The day is warm, with a gentle breeze,
and you can feel the Sun on your back …
The air is perfumed with the scent of freshly
mown grass and delicate flowers …

2. As you gather pace, you feel the path incline steeply …
Ahead is a mountain and you slowly begin to ascend.
The sides are steep and you must use all
your intuition to select the safest path …

3. Higher and higher you climb until you can see a plateau …
There is a fire burning in the middle of this flat ground,
its golden flames lapping the air …

4. By the fire is a pen and paper …
Stop, pick them up and think about a person(s)
to whom you have relinquished personal power …

5. Write the name(s) on the paper and hold it out to the flame …
Watch the fire eat the paper until it is utterly destroyed …

6. Bathe yourself in the warmth of the fire; feel its heat
regenerate your Solar Plexus, strengthening it …
Connect with the power of your Solar Plexus …
Know that you are a spiritual warrior and that you have the inner
resources and Divine guidance to help you overcome all life's challenges …

7. Revel in this moment of personal power and notice how it feels …
tune in to the signals that your body gives you so that you will recognize them again …

8. Now it's time to turn away from the flame,
climb down from the mountain and find the path again …
You are the same, but different …

9. Your power store is stronger and will become more so
every time you visit the flame on the mountain top …
And you can do so any time you choose.

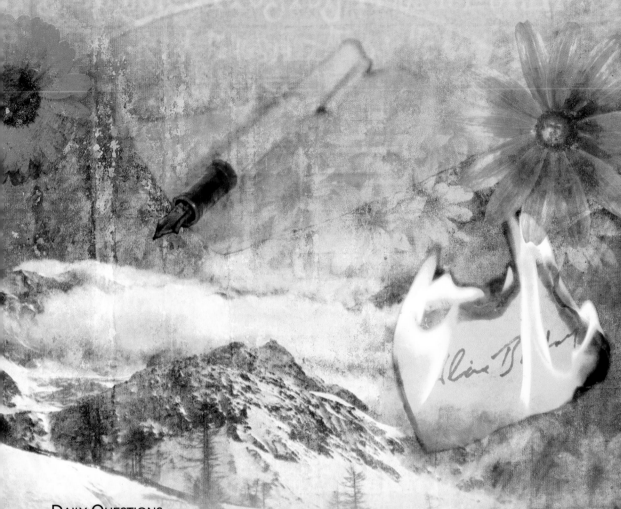

DAILY QUESTIONS

▽ What risks can you take to strengthen your personal power base? Consider confronting your fears about a particular person. How could you equalize your relationship with him/her?

▽ Have you recently acted subserviently? Did you gain anything? How can you prevent this happening again? Visualize a more empowering outcome.

▽ Who do you admire who "owns" themselves? How do they demonstrate personal power? How can you emulate them? If you admire a public figure, learn about them. When you are faced with a challenging decision, imagine what choice they would make.

▽ How do you use your anger? Controlled anger is a healthy expression of personal power. Practise giving vent to anger by punching a cushion.

AFFIRMATIONS

▽ I accept and value myself exactly as I am.

▽ I know I am becoming the best person I can be.

▽ I determine to treat myself with honour and respect.

▽ My personal power is becoming stronger each day.

▽ I am my own person. I choose how to think and behave.

▽ I deserve all the love, respect, joy, and prosperity that comes to me. I am open to receiving all life's good things.

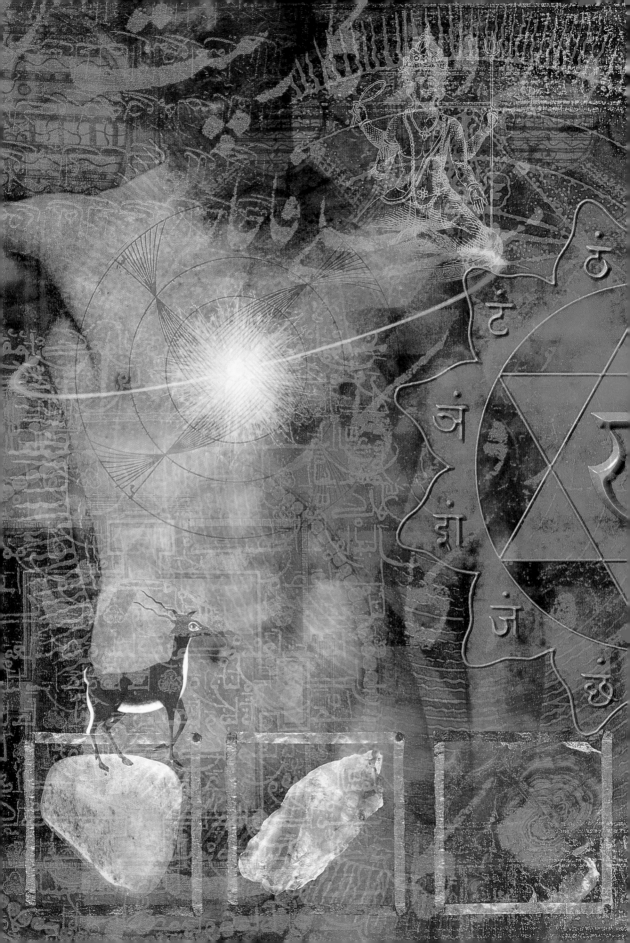

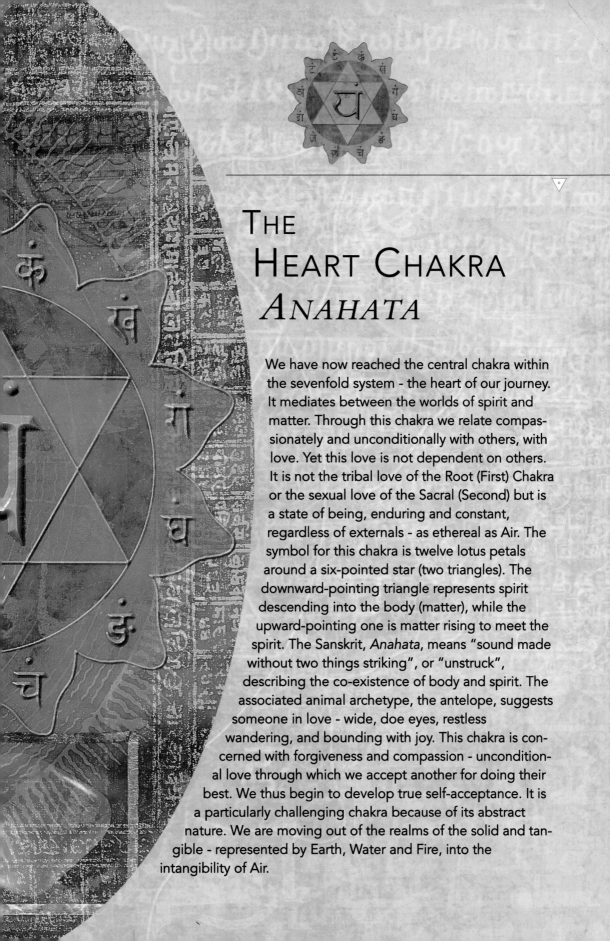

THE HEART CHAKRA
ANAHATA

We have now reached the central chakra within the sevenfold system - the heart of our journey. It mediates between the worlds of spirit and matter. Through this chakra we relate compassionately and unconditionally with others, with love. Yet this love is not dependent on others. It is not the tribal love of the Root (First) Chakra or the sexual love of the Sacral (Second) but is a state of being, enduring and constant, regardless of externals - as ethereal as Air. The symbol for this chakra is twelve lotus petals around a six-pointed star (two triangles). The downward-pointing triangle represents spirit descending into the body (matter), while the upward-pointing one is matter rising to meet the spirit. The Sanskrit, *Anahata*, means "sound made without two things striking", or "unstruck", describing the co-existence of body and spirit. The associated animal archetype, the antelope, suggests someone in love - wide, doe eyes, restless wandering, and bounding with joy. This chakra is concerned with forgiveness and compassion - unconditional love through which we accept another for doing their best. We thus begin to develop true self-acceptance. It is a particularly challenging chakra because of its abstract nature. We are moving out of the realms of the solid and tangible - represented by Earth, Water and Fire, into the intangibility of Air.

HEART CHAKRA CORRESPONDENCES

The chart for the Heart (Fourth) Chakra identifies the associations and symbolisms linked with the Fourth Chakra. As such it provides a "ready reference" of inspirations to use when assembling your altar arrangements (see pp.82-3) and crystal layouts (see pp.86-7). The chart will also help you with the various images you will need when composing your own meditations and visualizations. Incorporate as many of these symbols and themes as you feel is appropriate to your needs.

By reaquainting yourself regularly with this chakra as a prelude to the entire section on the Heart Chakra, you will help keep your mind focused on related issues, including an awareness of the opportunities for growth and development that come from forming loving relationships with others.

To make your chakra journey wholly successful and enjoyable you should prepare yourself by attending to certain practical requirements (see pp.25 and 87). Mastering the Heart Chakra helps us to enhance our emotional development and recognize the potency of that powerful energy we call "love".

CHAKRA CHARACTERISTICS

See which of the following characteristics of excessive ("too open"), deficient ("blocked"), and balanced chakra energy you can relate to - and then determine (should you choose) to take the necessary action, using the tools and techniques outlined in this chapter.

Too open (chakra spins too fast) - possessive, loves conditionally, witholds emotionally "to punish", overly dramatic
Blocked (chakra spins sluggishly or not at all) - fears rejection, loves too much, feels unworthy to receive love, self-pitying
Balanced (chakra maintains equilibrium and spins at correct vibrational speed) - compassionate, loves unconditionally, nurturing, desires spiritual experience in lovemaking

THE HEART CHAKRA

Sanskrit Name
Anahata

Meaning
Sound that is made without any two things striking; unstruck

Location
Centre of chest

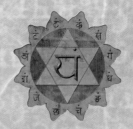

Symbol
Lotus of 12 petals, containing two intersecting circles that make up a 6-pointed star demonstrating the perfect balance between the downward-pointing spirit descending toward matter and the upward-pointing matter rising toward spirit.

Associated Colours
Green/pink

Element
Air

Ruling Planet
Venus

Archetypes
Functional - Lover
Dysfunctional - Performer

Associated Animal
Gazelle/antelope

Societal Association
Unconditional acceptance of others

Sacramental Association
Marriage

Emotional Dysfunctions
Co-dependency, melancholia, fears concerning loneliness, commitment and/or betrayal

Physical Dysfunctions
Shallow breathing, high blood pressure, heart disease, cancer

Associated Body Parts
Heart, chest, lungs, circulation

Glandular Connection
Thymus

Goals
Balance, compassion & self-acceptance

Associated Sense
Touch

Foods
Vegetables

Incense/Oils
Rose, Bergamot, Melissa

Crystals
Watermelon tourmaline, Rose quartz, Emerald, Green calcite, Jade, Azurite, Aventurine quartz, Malachite, Moonstone

Life Lesson
Forgiveness and compassion for oneself and others

Main Issue
Beliefs about love and relationships

Developmental Age
21-28 yrs

ARCHETYPES: HEART CHAKRA

The Heart (Fourth) Chakra further develops the internal focus that started with the lower chakras and is concerned with balancing the love of others and the love of ourselves. This central chakra is the passage through which we move from the lower to the higher centres, shifting us from the realm of basic needs into the realm of blessings. Our challenge is to pass the tests of unconditional love, compassion, and forgiveness with which we are challenged daily, in order to move on to the higher centres.

We tend to think of the heart as only concerned with "soft", irrational, feelings. We prefer to put greater emphasis on "head" activity, yet when allowed, the heart can be a far more accurate barometer of deeper needs. Listening to the heart in matters of love is vital to maintaining healthy, mutually respectful, relationships. As we make our journey toward the Higher Self our relationships painfully expose us to how little we love ourselves. When we strip away the thin veneer that covers lack of self-intimacy and fill it energetically with joy, peace, and self-acceptance, we start to build the solid foundation upon which unconditional love flourishes. Those who dismiss or shun intimacy demonstrate their fear of looking inward. They neglect the opportunities that relationships offer for self-knowledge - acknowledging and loving our dark side as well as the parts we admire. This is the basis of unconditional love.

The negative archetype associated with the Heart Chakra is the Performer. Such people mask personal wounds by playing at being "in love"; a very different experience to truly loving someone. Their way is a theoretical, cerebral, activity, without putting heart and soul into the relationship. True Lovers, on the other hand, have the capacity to love themselves unconditionally. Because they don't need other people to buoy them up, they freely open their hearts and share self-acceptance with others. These generous, free-spirited, individuals offer themselves wholeheartedly to others because they know that the core of their being is secure. Being in touch

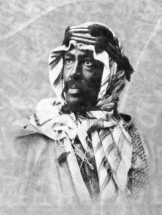

LOVING TOO MUCH

So often we profess to love another person but we wrap the love up in a cloak of jealousy, possessiveness, and emotional instability. We may misinterpret the strong feelings engendered by these dysfunctional attitudes for "love" when the experience is really about externalizing something that needs to come from within, in order to avoid facing up to long-held fears concerning hurt and betrayal.

with their emotions, they take a lighter approach to relationships, in the certain knowledge that the forgiveness and compassion, which their dysfunctional counterparts look to others to provide, is available to them internally at any time.

THE LOVER

Lovers are magnetic, radiant individuals who truly "own" themselves. They are easily recognizable because it is impossible not to be affected by their positive energy.

THE PERFORMER

A common example of this personality is the co-dependent, who looks outside for the love they crave, kidding themselves that their wounds can be healed by finding someone else to draw strength from. However, fear of betrayal, one of the emotional dysfunctions of the Heart Chakra, sabotages any chance of real happiness with another.

By undertaking the meditation, daily questions, and affirmations on pages 88-9, you will be able to cast aside the "theory" of loving and assume the self-ownership of the true Lover.

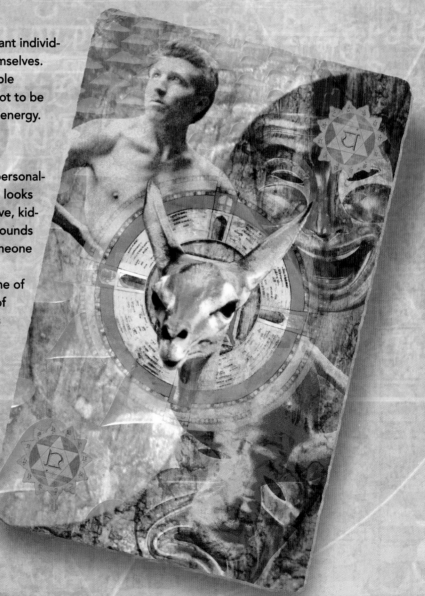

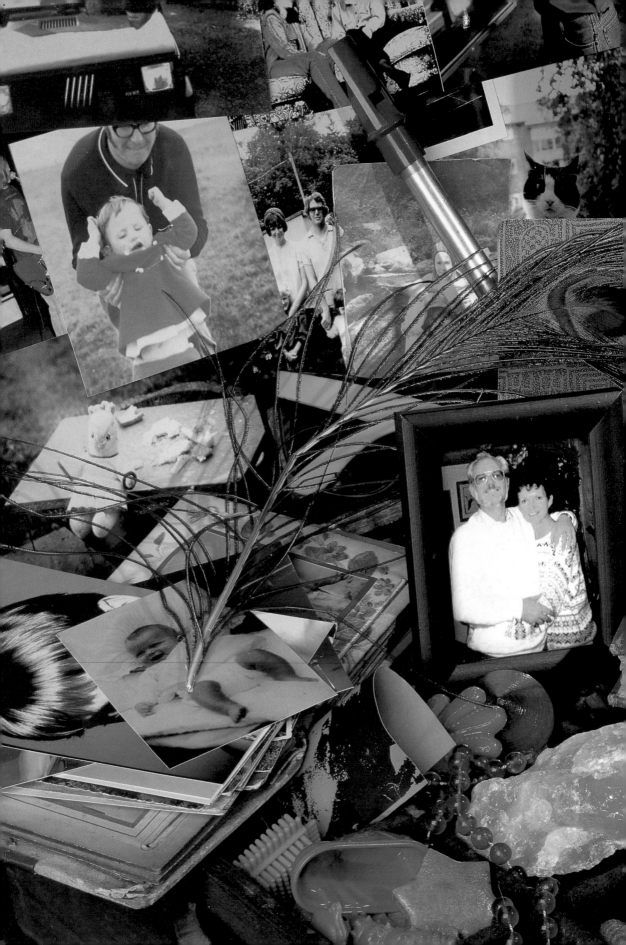

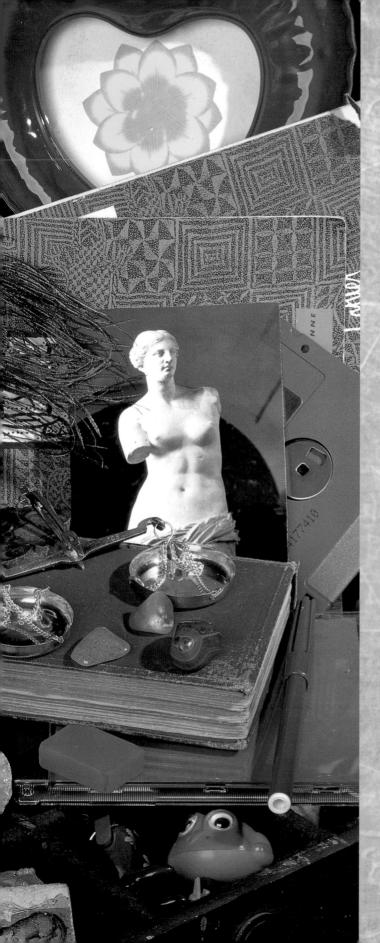

ALTAR:
HEART CHAKRA

These nineteen-year-old twin girls were distraught when their father left their mother. They felt hatred, jealousy, fear, despair, and betrayal. They knew their parents had been unhappy, but found it difficult not to blame their father and despise their mother. A favourite aunt suggested they create an altar to the Heart Chakra, to encourage compassion and forgiveness. They determined to love both parents equally for their fallibilities and their strengths. This led them to think of how they failed to love themselves for all their qualities - "good" and "bad".

▽ Picture of their relations, to remind them of support beyond immediate family
▽ Green-hued peacock feather, representing the 4th chakra symbols of flight and air
▽ Small scales denoting balance (love and hate)
▽ Green beads and tumble stones
▽ A postcard of Botticelli's *Venus*, Goddess of Love
▽ Green pen to maintain written communication with their father
▽ Rose quartz, symbol of love
▽ Green-covered journals for recording their feelings
▽ Book on developing self-love
▽ Pictures of their parents
▽ Twelve-petalled lotus in a heart-shaped frame

This altar is the twins' attempt to work on the Heart Chakra. It is a case study, for inspiration. Choose objects which have personal significance for you.

EXERCISES: HEART CHAKRA

Given the dual nature of the Heart Chakra in prompting us to focus both on loving ourselves and loving others, it should come as no surprise that these are exercises for this area which can be done alone or with someone else. Be aware of the need to ensure that your partner really wants to take part in the Heart Connection Exercise, and is not persuaded into it out of a sense of obligation.

1. Lie face down on the floor with your arms by your sides, palms facing toward your hips. Breath in, imagining a string attached to your hands pulling upward on to your lower back and lifting your upper body away from the floor. Keep your neck elongated as you look straight ahead, breathing smoothly. Maintain the pose for as long as possible.

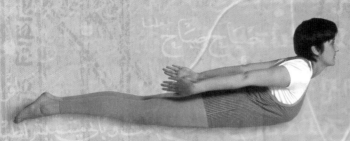

2. Lower yourself gently to the floor again and, as you breathe in, extend your arms out at shoulder level like wings and lift your upper body away from the floor - again facing forward. Imagine your heart area opening up and being offered as a gift to an imaginary recipient in front of you. Ensure that your shoulders don't hunch up, so that you allow your neck to lengthen.

3. A third variation on this exercise is, from Position 1, to breathe in and lift your upper body off the floor, at the same time extending your arms directly in front of you. If it feels more comfortable lift your straight legs away from the floor also. Visualize your heart opening, ensuring that you don't hold your breath or tense your muscles. Then lower your arms and legs to the floor on exhalation.

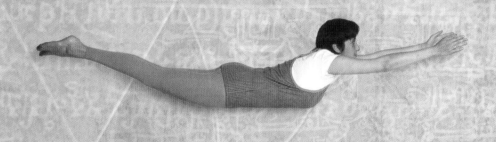

HEART CONNECTION EXERCISE

This exercise is good for developing mutual unconditional love. Lay your right hands on each other's Heart Chakra and your left over the other's hand. Gaze into each other's eyes for a few minutes. Then close your eyes for a while, sensing a continuing deep connection.

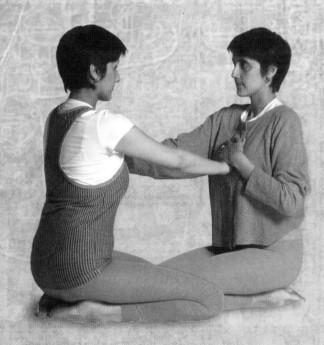

KEY CRYSTALS: HEART CHAKRA

Crystals that are useful to use on the Heart Chakra vary between the commonly associated colour pink, for "love", and green. The latter, particularly, is traditionally regarded as a psychologically balancing colour, apt not just for the equilibrium of physical, mental, and emotional energies but also the balance between giving and receiving love. (See also pp.26-7 for information on Crystal Healing.)

ROSE QUARTZ

The soothing vibration of this gentle pink Quartz helps comfort anyone suffering from emotional "wounds". It prompts the development of self-love, through which one can learn to love others unconditionally. The loving energy of Rose quartz also helps you become more receptive to the joys of all forms of creative endeavour.

GREEN JADE

This crystal is said to offer reassurance and protection to those feeling vulnerable, when placed over the Heart Chakra. Its gentle resonance encourages strength and stability when you feel afraid or threatened. Green is the energy of balance and healing and light green Jade carries a vibration of love and forgiveness.

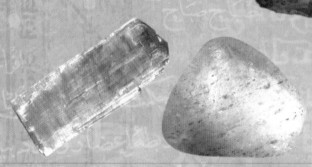

AVENTURINE QUARTZ

Most commonly green, Aventurine contains particles of Mica or Hematite, giving it a metallic glint. This uplifting crystal is good for depression, encouraging lightness and enthusiasm for life. It is valuable in maintaining the balance of the Heart Chakra after it has been closed down by grief, and generally protects this area.

WATERMELON TOURMALINE

This Tourmaline usually has a green rind and pink centre. It is said to be the "superactivator" of the Heart Chakra, allowing this area to become connected with the Higher Self. Watermelon tourmaline helps with any emotional dysfunction and enhances co-operative efforts and tact.

GREEN CALCITE

This crystal helps to develop the strength needed to cope with change or transition, by forming a link between the heart and the head. It is an excellent choice when dealing with emotional "wounds" affecting the heart and encourages compassion and tenderness toward oneself and others.

The Twins (see also pp.82-3)

The twins preferred to wear a piece of crystal jewellery rather than have a full body layout. One chose a pale Jade heart and the other two plain Jade rings and wore them over the Heart area. Each morning the girls engaged in a ritual in front of their altar in which they imagined the soft, green energy of the Jade calming their broken hearts, helping them achieve an inner serenity and balanced perspective on their circumstances. At night the pendants were placed under their pillows, as in Mayan culture Jade was used to release suppressed emotions during dreaming.

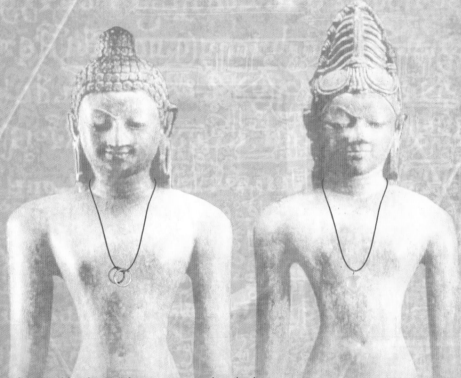

Approach crystal healing with an open mind and take the time to choose and position crystals with your needs and wishes uppermost.

▽ *Choose a warm, comfortable place.*

▽ *Ensure you are not going to be disturbed.*

▽ *Play gentle music or nature sounds.*

▽ *Burn incense or scented candles.*

▽ *Wear loose clothes.*

▽ *Go to the bathroom first.*

▽ *Have a glass of water to rehydrate and ground you afterwards.*

▽ *Cleanse and tune the crystals (see p.27).*

MEDITATION: HEART CHAKRA

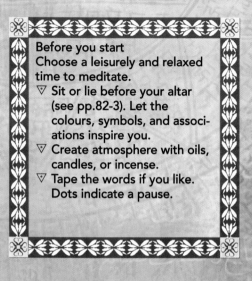

Before you start
Choose a leisurely and relaxed time to meditate.
▽ Sit or lie before your altar (see pp.82-3). Let the colours, symbols, and associations inspire you.
▽ Create atmosphere with oils, candles, or incense.
▽ Tape the words if you like. Dots indicate a pause.

1. You are beginning a journey to the Heart Chakra ...
Are you nervous, excited, pained? Acknowledge these feelings, but don't dwell on them ...
Know that you are safe, protected - loved ...

2. See yourself on a red pathway.
Feel firm earth beneath your feet ...
Notice the road changing to sandy orange, then rippling beneath your feet like water. Your feet seem lighter and help you move closer to your destination ...

3. The road changes again, to a rich golden yellow ...
Feel its warmth penetrate your feet, warming your entire being ...
Everything is bathed in golden sunlight ...

4. Look ahead and see that the road has become green and leads to a pink castle ... As you take this green pathway it falls away beneath you, as if you were walking on air ... You are now at the entrance of the pink castle.

5. Feel the heavy door swing open into a vast pink hall ... On a plinth lies your heart. How does it look? Is it frozen in a block of ice? Or encased in chains? Or is it haemorrhaging energy from being too open to others ... Consider its state ... Don't judge what you see - you are here to heal it ...

6. Have the appropriate remedy available to you. Take a pick and chip away at the ice, breathing warm air to melt it faster ... Unlock the chains with a golden key from your pocket ... Watch as your heart expands in freedom ...

7. Place your hands lovingly on any scars and send Universal Love to your heart to dissolve them ...
Allow your natural healing energy to give your heart what it needs.

8. Notice how your heart responds positively to this attention ... Be aware of a connection between what is in your mind's eye and what is going on in your body ... Enjoy these moments ...

9. Caress your heart and send it limitless Universal Love, knowing that the more it receives the more love will be available to others.

DAILY QUESTIONS

▽ Do you respond to others through the mind and intellect rather than the Heart? Tune in to your Heart's message. Focus on what you truly feel, without judging. The Heart has the answers.

▽ How much do you feel connected with others? Try going out and smiling at people. You'll be surprised how many smile back.

▽ Are you hard on yourself for "failing"? This chakra is about balance - not just with others but with yourself. Honour your dark and light sides.

▽ Do you "put on a good face"? Learn to detach from your feelings. When your heart is full of pain, acknowledge that it represents another lesson. Rejoice and move forward.

▽ Are you compassionate, or do you judge others? Everyone's reality is different. Know that no-one can hurt you - it's how you react to what they do to you that is the cause of your pain.

AFFIRMATIONS

▽ I send love to everyone I know; all hearts are open to receive my love.

▽ I accept that pain is an essential part of my growth and development.

▽ I love myself for who I am and the potential within me.

▽ All past hurt I release into the hands of love.

▽ I am grateful for all the love that is in my life.

▽ Other people deserve my compassion.

▽ The love I feel for myself and others is unconditional.

▽ Love will set me free. Others love the best they can. If someone doesn't love me "enough", they may be limited in their expression of love and deserve my compassion.

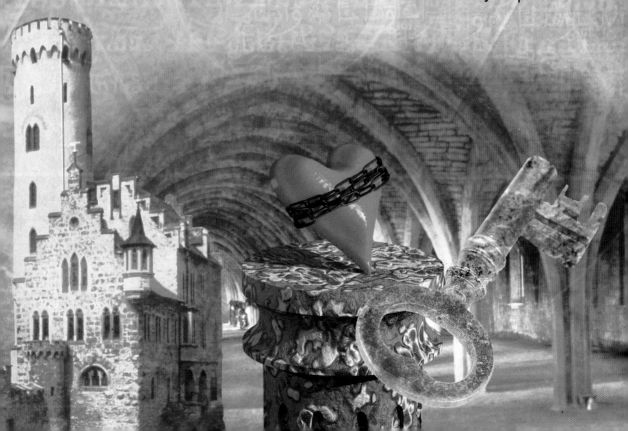

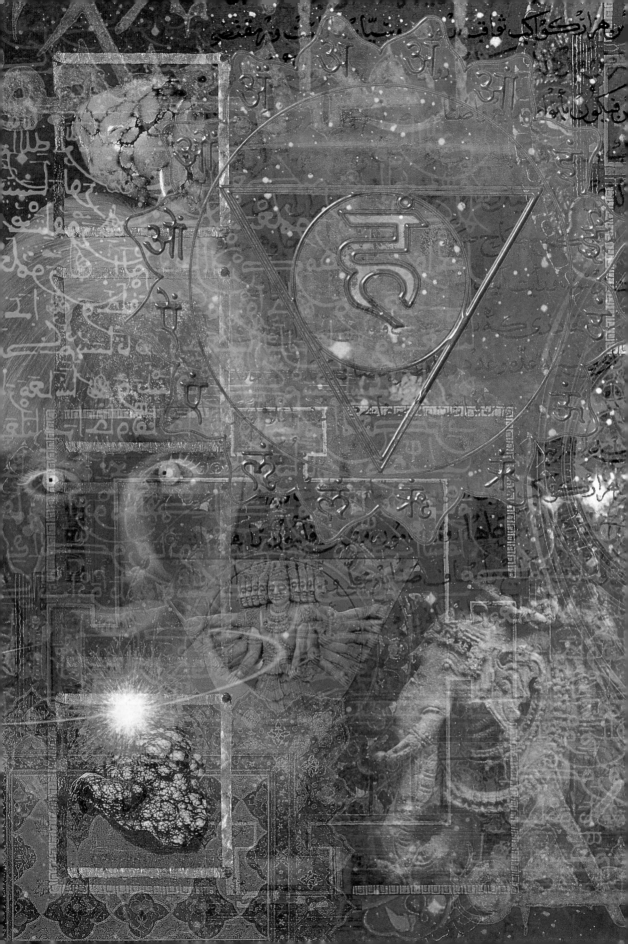

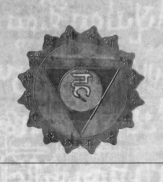

THE
THROAT CHAKRA
VISHUDDHA

The Throat Chakra is the first of the higher centres - associated with communication, self-expression, and creativity through sound. The Sanskrit, *Vishuddha* - "purification" - offers a clue to this type of communication: not everyday chatter but purposeful thoughts and speech. It is about personal expression combined with responsibility. Developing the Throat Chakra means choosing words that bring value to communication. A further implication of Vishuddha is that only by successfully working through the lower four chakras can you reach the purification necessary to open the Throat Chakra, which resonates to the colour blue in its less intense shades.

The Hindu symbol of Vishuddha is a lotus of 16 petals containing the Sanskrit vowels, thought to represent spirit. Within the lotus is a triangle symbolizing speech and a full Moon and Airavata, the many-tusked elephant. In addition to sound, this chakra is connected with hearing. It is a sad fact that active listening is neglected today and we need to develop the outer ear before the subtle inner ear can be available to us. Those who operate from the higher chakras frequently find the real message behind their words is not "heard". When the Throat Chakra is functioning thought and speech slow down and communication is more considered.

THROAT CHAKRA CORRESPONDENCES

This chart for the Throat (Fifth) Chakra identifies all the associations and symbolisms linked with this particular chakra. As such it provides a "ready reference" of inspirations to use when you carry out practical exercises such as assembling your altar arrangements (see pp.96-7) or choosing appropriate stones for crystal work (see pp.100-1). This chart will also help you with the various images you will need when composing your meditations and visualizations. Incorporate as many of these symbols and themes as you feel is appropriate to your needs.

By reacquainting yourself regularly with this chakra chart as a prelude to the section on the Throat Chakra, you will help to keep your mind focused on related issues, including the importance of expressing your emotions and communicating your truth to yourself and others.

To make your chakra journey successful and enjoyable you should prepare yourself by attending to certain practical requirements (see pp.25 and 101). Mastering the Throat Chakra helps us grasp the importance of purifying ourselves by honestly recognizing how we feel and having the confidence to communicate those emotions to others.

CHAKRA CHARACTERISTICS
See which of the following characteristics of excessive ("too open"), deficient ("blocked"), and balanced chakra energy you can relate to - and then determine (should you choose) to take the necessary action, using the tools and techniques outlined in this chapter.

Too open (chakra spins too fast) - over-talkative, dogmatic, self-righteous, arrogant
Blocked (chakra spins sluggishly or not at all) - holds back from self-expression, unreliable, holds inconsistent views
Balanced (chakra maintains equilibrium and spins at correct vibrational speed) - good communicator, contented, finds it easy to meditate, artistically inspired

THE THROAT CHAKRA

Sanskrit Name
Vishuddha

Meaning
Purification

Location
Centrally, at base of neck

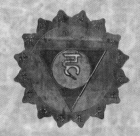

Symbol
Lotus with 16 petals, containing a downward-pointing triangle within which is a circle representing the full Moon.

Associated Colour
Blue

Element
Ether

Ruling Planet
Mercury

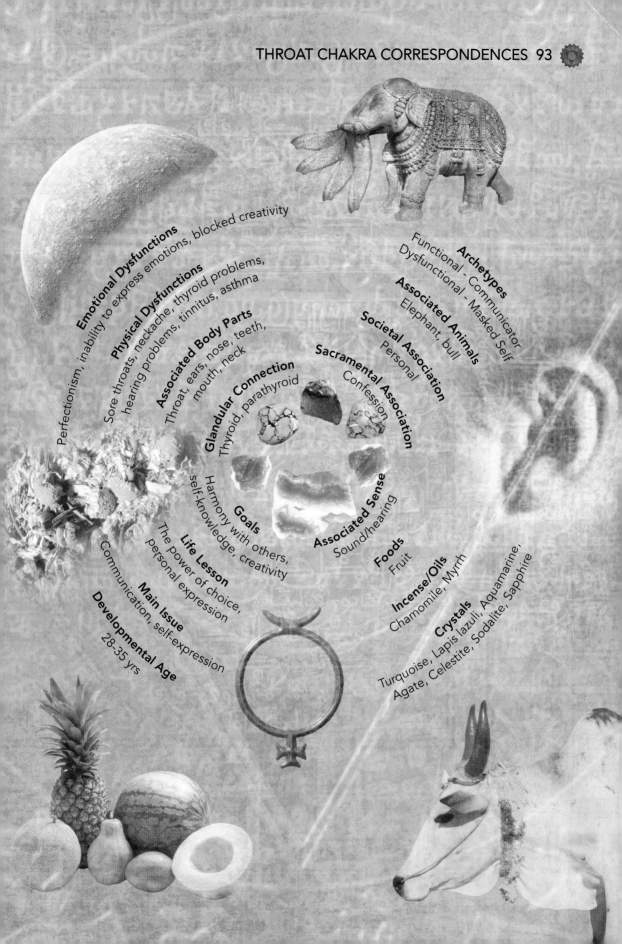

Archetypes
Functional - Communicator
Dysfunctional - Masked Self

Associated Animals
Elephant, bull

Societal Association
Personal

Sacramental Association
Confession

Associated Sense
Sound/hearing

Foods
Fruit

Incense/Oils
Chamomile, Myrrh

Crystals
Turquoise, Lapis lazuli, Aquamarine,
Agate, Celestite, Sodalite, Sapphire

Emotional Dysfunctions
Perfectionism, inability to express emotions, blocked creativity

Physical Dysfunctions
Sore throats, neckache, thyroid problems,
hearing problems, tinnitus, asthma

Associated Body Parts
Throat, ears, nose, teeth,
mouth, neck

Glandular Connection
Thyroid, parathyroid

Goals
Harmony with others,
self-knowledge, creativity

Life Lesson
The power of choice,
personal expression

Main Issue
Communication, self-expression

Developmental Age
28-35 yrs

ARCHETYPES: THROAT CHAKRA

The next time you meet someone who appears to have trouble expressing themselves, see if their chin is held down on the chest, hiding the throat area in a childlike manner. This shows that this person is vulnerable in the Throat (Fifth) Chakra. Such people have frequently to clear the throat because esoterically it is being choked by the truths they are having to swallow. They may speak in an unexpectedly dull, monotonous tone. They may attempt to contribute to group discussions, but because of inarticulateness or lack of enthusiasm they are frequently not "heard" by others. These are all clues to a dysfunctional Throat Chakra.

In its extreme form the negative archetype associated with the Throat Chakra is the Masked Self. Here we have someone incapable of openly and honestly expressing feelings. They may wish to refuse an unreasonable (or reasonable) request, but say "yes" anyway. Anger and frustration then builds up, further blocking the Throat Chakra, which may manifest itself physically as sore throat, glandular fever, stiff neck, and thyroid problems. The silence is not of lack of communication but lack of truthful expression.

By contrast, Communicators "walk their talk'. They often have wonderful speaking voices which others delight in listening to and may have chosen jobs in the areas of public speaking, teaching, broadcasting, personal development training, and various therapies. That is not to say that all who work in these fields are true Communicators - but the ones who excel undoubtedly do so because they express themselves with amazing clarity and purpose. It is the congruence that listeners sense between their self-expression and sincerity of the inner Self that makes Communicators so compelling. Both spoken and written words are uttered in a considered way and are hardly ever peppered with inanities or profanities.

Communicators recognize their right to express their hurt or anger, but do so in such a way that it doesn't diminish the other person. They integrate both heart and mind in their communications with others. They also recognize the power of the spoken and written word and, by taking responsibility for their feelings, do not abuse them.

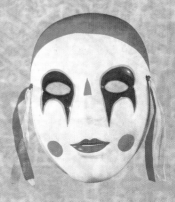

THE PAIN OF THE MASKED SELF

This pain is often caused by childhood traumas when the Masked Self was brought up to be "seen and not heard", frequently told to "shut up", and made to feel that their opinions were worthless. In order to cope with this rejection of their true Self they suppressed it. That sad child remains locked in adult form, choosing to neglect responsibility for growing up and taking charge of life.

THE COMMUNICATOR

Having worked through their lower chakras and achieved the compassion required of the Heart, Communicators know that if others don't "hear" what they have to say this is not an indictment of their communicative abilities but merely demonstrates that the recipient is not yet at a stage when they can take on board what is being said.

THE MASKED SELF

Sometimes the Masked Self appears as a clown; someone who is always laughing, making jokes, and taking an unrealistically positive view of any situation. In reality they are putting on the mask of comedy in an attempt to hide the tragedy of feeling that no-one loves or will listen to them.

Try out the meditation, daily questions, and affirmations on pages 102-3 to give confidence to your Masked Self and set free your Communicator.

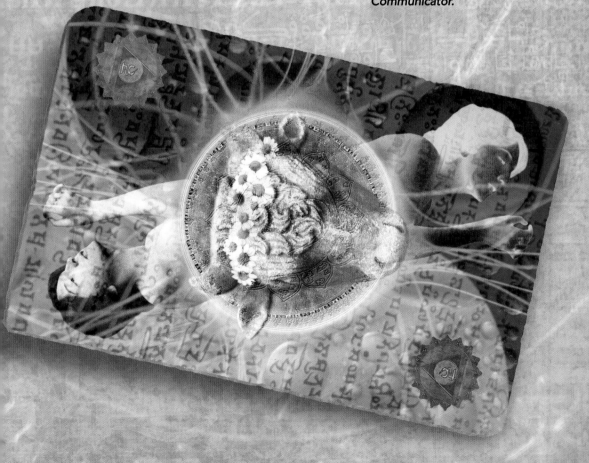

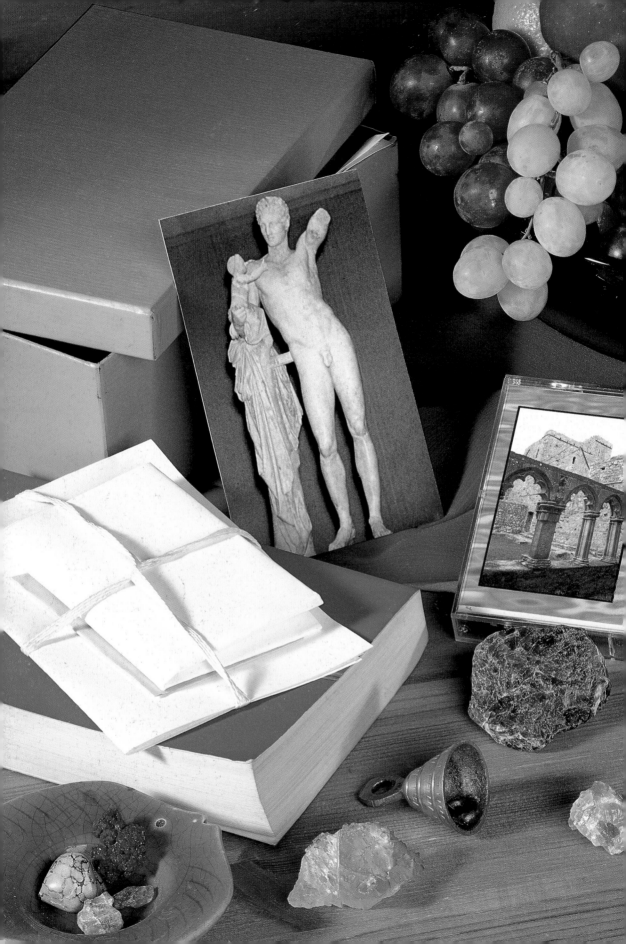

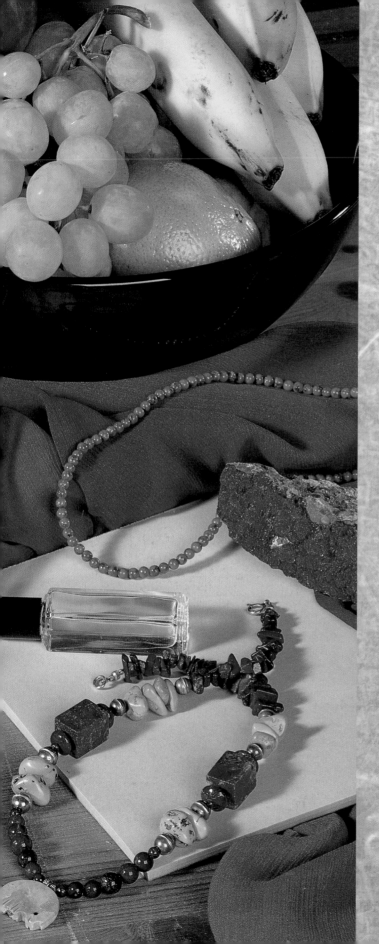

ALTAR:
THROAT CHAKRA

Sarah's job in administration had never fulfilled her. She had excelled at creative writing at school and had wanted to become a journalist, but she had never managed to express her wishes and had drifted into her present office job. She realized that this was also due to her belief that her work was not good enough. She had been brought up in a family where to even acknowledge one's talents was frowned upon. This had caused her constantly to undermine herself. After a friend reassured her that she had a real talent, Sarah decided to focus on allowing her creativity to flow more freely; also to develop communication skills, to bring her abilities to the attention of others. This she did by setting up an altar:

▽ A bright turquoise and blue cloth
▽ Native American Lapis lazuli and Turquoise necklaces
▽ Small brass bell representing sound and resonance
▽ A collection of her own poems and short stories in a blue box
▽ Favourite tape of chants
▽ Picture of Hermes, messenger of the Gods
▽ Bowl of fruit
▽ Bottle of white musk
▽ Hand-written affirmations celebrating her successful creative endeavours
▽ A book given her at school as a prize for creative writing
▽

This altar is Sarah's attempt to work on the Throat Chakra. It is a case study, for inspiration. Choose objects which have personal significance for you.

Exercise: Throat Chakra

For most of us the neck tends to be one of the areas in which we suffer from stiffness and tension, as a result of stress and poor posture. Esoterically this area is the bridge between which the energetic flow connecting the mind and body is channelled. If this flow is hindered in any way stagnancy and blockages occur which also contribute to rigidity in the neck area. The following inverted yoga poses - two variations on the same theme - help loosen the neck area and in particular stimulate the thyroid gland associated with the Throat Chakra.

Shoulder Stand

If you feel confident, do the shoulder stand directly on the floor or mat. Lie flat. Bend your knees with your feet flat on the floor so the heels are close to your buttocks. Lift your lower back slightly and, bringing your knees toward your head, swing your trunk and legs up - at the same time moving your hands to support your lower back. Stretch your legs so that they are straight above you. Be aware of your breath, inhaling and exhaling slowly through your nose. Hold this pose as long as is comfortable.

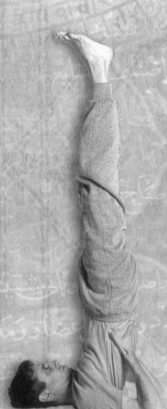

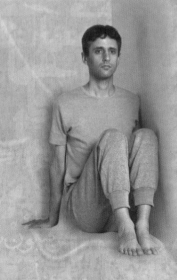

1. If you feel you need more support, use a wall to rest your legs against. Start off by sitting right next to the wall.

2. Raise your legs so that they are flat against the wall and lie back with your buttocks against this solid surface.

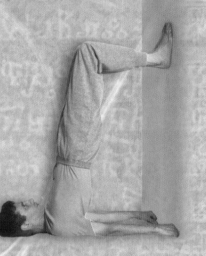

3. Bend your legs at the knees, pressing your feet flat against the wall and raise your hips and chest.

4. Support your lower back with your hands, keeping your elbows close to your body. Straighten your legs, keeping your feet on the wall, at the same time lifting your chest, abdomen, and hips away from it. Breathing evenly through the nose, relax in this position for several minutes.

KEY CRYSTALS: THROAT CHAKRA

A major theme of the Throat Chakra is communication in all its forms, and this is achieved by the use of crystals of varying shades of blue. There are many suitable choices, so be guided by your intuition and select stones with which you have a personal affinity, rather than feel you are being dictated to in your choice. (See also pp.26-7 for information on Crystal Healing.)

LAPIS LAZULI

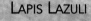

A deep-blue crystal with gold or white flecks. Another stone of self-expression and artistic enterprise, Lapis helps expand your awareness and intellectual capacity. Its energizing effect on the Throat Chakra helps activate a new realm of consciousness and the mental clarity necessary to communicate this effectively to others.

TURQUOISE

This beautiful crystal helps stimulate the Throat Chakra so that you can articulate emotional issues. It is wonderful to use when involved in creative endeavours, as it helps link intuitive inspiration with all self-expression. Turquoise is said to help you find your true path in life by attunement with the Higher Self.

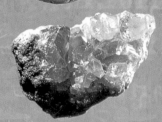

CELESTITE

A soft and fragile crystal used by Bengali priests to colour flames in order to impress followers. This is a useful stone for mental activity since it can help you take on board complex ideas and re-transmit them simply. Said to assist in clairaudience and dream recall, Celestite can add another dimension if you have stories to tell.

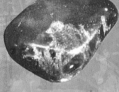

SODALITE

Loosely resembling Lapis lazuli, this crystal occurs in various shades of blue, as well as other colours. It encourages objectivity and new perspectives and brings about a harmony between the conscious and unconscious minds. Sodalite helps you to recognize and articulate your true feelings and shows how to move forward in life with a lightness of heart.

AQUAMARINE

A crystal that is suitable for anyone in the deadline-driven media business, since is has a calming, stress-reducing effect, particularly when you need to communicate to large audiences. Aquamarine enables you to assimilate knowledge, not just about the world at large but about yourself. It stimulates and cleanses the Throat Chakra, elevating any communication beyond the mundane.

SARAH (see also pp.96-7)
All the blue crystals described here (see left)
were used to help Sarah in her desire to
express her talents both verbally and in written form. Stones were positioned on and
around the Throat Chakra and Sarah
visualized the blue energy creating an open
pathway between her throat and her mind.
Advised by her crystal healer, Sarah acquired
a traditional Native American Turquoise and
Lapis lazuli necklace, which nestled on her
lower throat area. She regularly wore it while
writing and found she could tap in to her
innate creativity much more easily. This included the ability to write compelling letters to
prospective commissioning editors in order to
bring her writing talents to the attention of a
wider audience.

Approach crystal healing with an open mind and
take the time to choose and position crystals with
your needs and wishes uppermost.
▽ Choose a warm, comfortable place.
▽ Ensure you are not going to be disturbed.
▽ Play gentle music or nature sounds.
▽ Burn incense or scented candles.
▽ Wear loose clothes.
▽ Go to the bathroom first.
▽ Have a glass of water to rehydrate and ground
   you afterwards.
▽ Cleanse and tune the crystals (see p.27).

MEDITATION: THROAT CHAKRA

Before you start
Choose a leisurely and relaxed time to meditate.
▽ Sit or lie before your altar (see pp.96-7). Let the colours, symbols, and associations inspire you.
▽ Create atmosphere with oils, candles, or incense.
▽ Tape the words if you like. Dots indicate a pause.

1. Take up a comfortable position and breathe slowly and deeply through your nose.

2. Tense each set of muscles in turn, from feet to your head …
feel yourself sink heavily into the floor or chair …

3. Now focus on your lower head and neck and imagine a beautiful blue mist washing inside your mouth … bathing your throat cavity … swirling around your ears … caressing your neck … gliding over your tongue … relaxing your jaw … so that the area becomes supple and free …

4. Be aware of any tension and draw the attention of this blue mist to that area so it can be released by it …

5. Be aware of your breathing and allow each inhalation to increase the intensity of the blue mist … each exhalation to spread this blue mist throughout your throat, mouth, tongue, ears and neck … strengthening each area … allowing you to speak your truth … to express your feelings honestly, openly, with compassion to yourself and others …

6. As you continue to sense the blue mist swirling around your Throat Chakra think of the words "I want" and "I need" … What do you want?… What do you need? … You have the right to ask for what you want and what you need … you have the right to have your demands listened to with respect and patience …

7. Determine to speak out for yourself in some way every day …

8. Know that by meditating on this beautiful mist daily you will strengthen and support your Throat Chakra and move toward a time when your needs and wants are listened to … and met … Because you have within you everything you need to meet those needs for yourself … And by accepting this you will find that others will support and honour them.

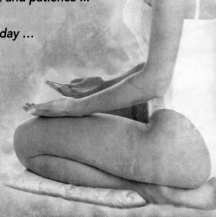

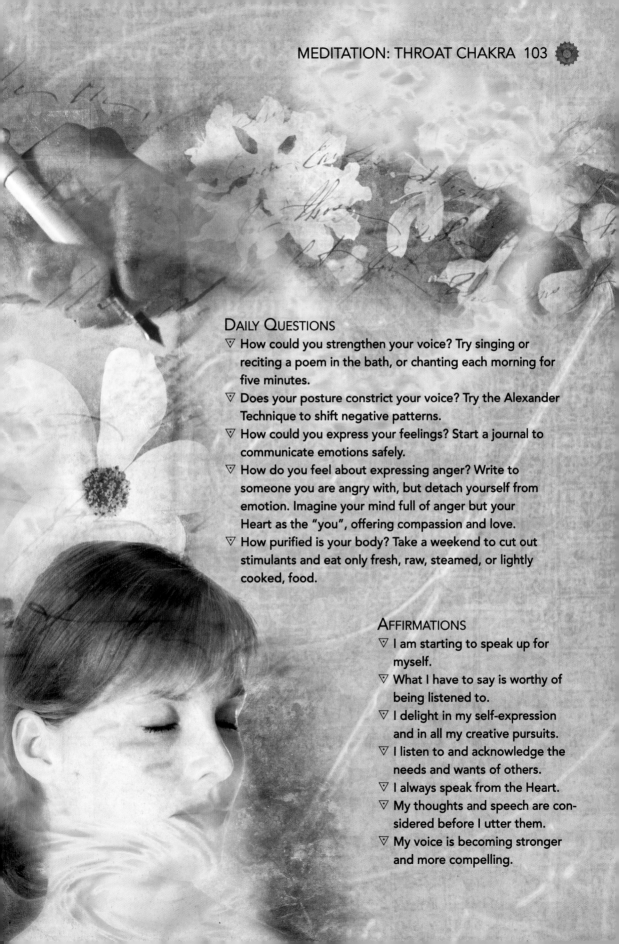

DAILY QUESTIONS

▽ How could you strengthen your voice? Try singing or reciting a poem in the bath, or chanting each morning for five minutes.

▽ Does your posture constrict your voice? Try the Alexander Technique to shift negative patterns.

▽ How could you express your feelings? Start a journal to communicate emotions safely.

▽ How do you feel about expressing anger? Write to someone you are angry with, but detach yourself from emotion. Imagine your mind full of anger but your Heart as the "you", offering compassion and love.

▽ How purified is your body? Take a weekend to cut out stimulants and eat only fresh, raw, steamed, or lightly cooked, food.

AFFIRMATIONS

▽ I am starting to speak up for myself.

▽ What I have to say is worthy of being listened to.

▽ I delight in my self-expression and in all my creative pursuits.

▽ I listen to and acknowledge the needs and wants of others.

▽ I always speak from the Heart.

▽ My thoughts and speech are considered before I utter them.

▽ My voice is becoming stronger and more compelling.

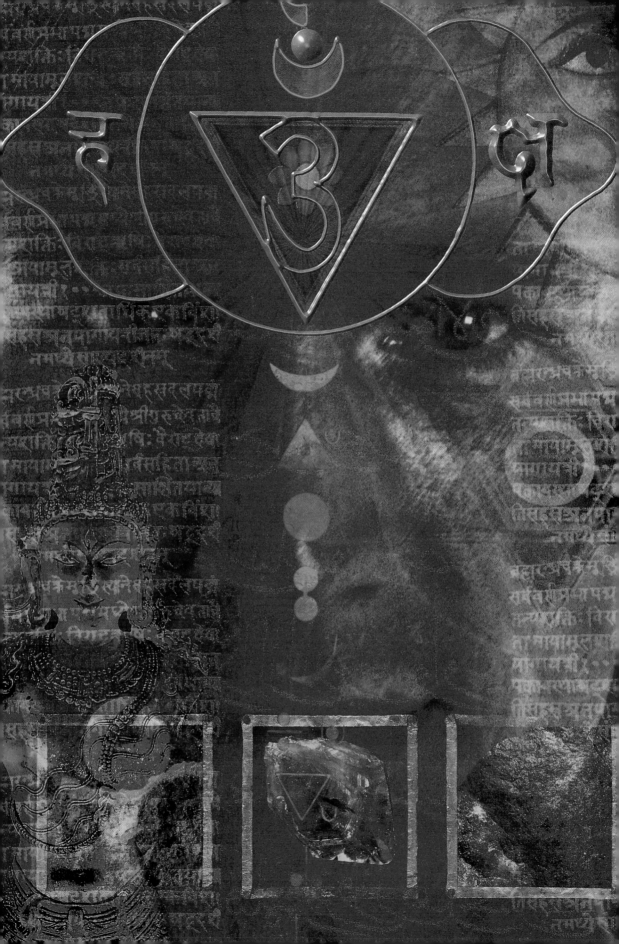

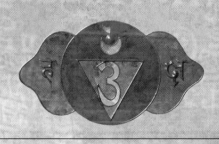

THE THIRD EYE CHAKRA

AJNA

The penultimate chakra on our journey through the sevenfold chakra system is *Ajna*, meaning "to perceive", "to know", and also "to control". Our physical eyes are the tools with which we perceive tangibles, while the Sixth Chakra - the "third eye", above and between the eyebrows - offers us the ability to intuit things for which we have no concrete evidence. In everyday terms we talk about "hunches" when we "know" things we cannot rationalize. Often we choose to be blind to the potential illuminated by our Third Eye. In its connection with the higher functions of consciousness, the Third Eye Chakra is a psychic tool reminding us that everything we see, hear, smell, touch, or taste started as an inner vision or "in-sight". The symbol of this chakra is the two-petalled lotus, like wings either side of a circle, within which is a downward-pointing triangle. The petals are like our two eyes each side of the Third Eye; the two sides of the brain working in harmony; or wings transcending physical limitations; and the two worlds of reality - manifest and unmanifest. The non-physical nature of this chakra is represented by Light. In the physical sense Light hits the eyes and is translated into images. In the realm of the esoteric, intuition is like a light coming on in the brain and may be accompanied by an internal image. These are our "eureka" moments.

THIRD EYE CHAKRA CORRESPONDENCES

This chart for the Third Eye (Sixth) Chakra identifies all the associations and symbolisms linked with this particular chakra. As such it provides a "ready reference" of inspirations to use when you carry out practical exercises such as assembling your altar arrangements (see pp.110-11) or choosing appropriate stones for crystal work (see pp.114-15). This chart will also help you with the various images you will need when composing your own meditations and visualizations. Incorporate as many of these symbols and themes as you feel is appropriate to your personal needs.

By reacquainting yourself regularly with this chakra chart as a prelude to the section on the Third Eye Chakra, you will help to keep your mind focused on related issues, including the awareness of the benefits to be gained from transcending the purely physical world and opening yourself up to intuitive sight and wisdom. It allows you to tap in to the limitless knowledge which you can access directly in order to answer the questions for which you tend to look to others - be they mentors, gurus, therapists, astrologers, or psychics - to satisfy.

CHAKRA CHARACTERISTICS

See which of the following characteristics of excessive ("too open"), deficient ("blocked"), and balanced chakra energy you can relate to - and then determine (should you choose) to take the necessary action, using the tools and techniques outlined in this chapter.

Too open (chakra spins too fast) - highly logical, dogmatic, authoritarian, arrogant
Blocked (chakra spins sluggishly or not at all) - undisciplined, fears success, tendency toward schizophrenia, sets sights too low
Balanced (chakra maintains equilibrium and spins at correct vibrational speed) - charismatic, highly intuitive, not attached to material things, may experience unusual phenomena

THE THIRD EYE CHAKRA

Sanskrit Name
Ajna

Meaning
To perceive, to know

Location
Above & between eyebrows

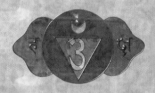

Symbol
Lotus with 2 large petals on either side, resembling eyes or wings, around a circle containing a downward-pointing triangle

Associated Colour
Indigo

Element
Light/Telepathic energy

Ruling Planets
Neptune, Jupiter

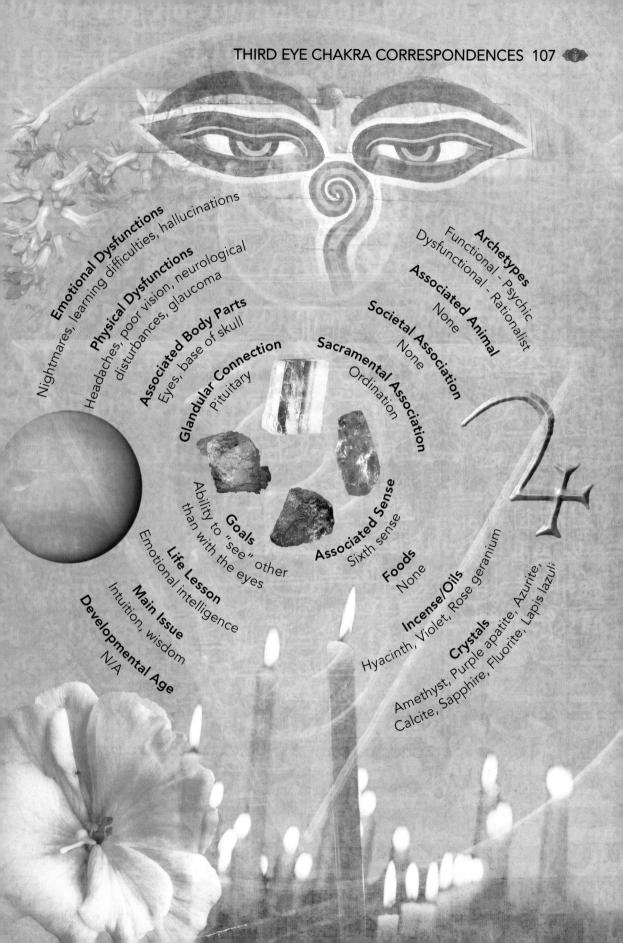

Emotional Dysfunctions
Nightmares, learning difficulties, hallucinations

Physical Dysfunctions
Headaches, poor vision, neurological disturbances, glaucoma

Associated Body Parts
Eyes, base of skull

Glandular Connection
Pituitary

Goals
Ability to "see" other than with the eyes

Life Lesson
Emotional intelligence

Main Issue
Intuition, wisdom

Developmental Age
N/A

Archetypes
Functional - Psychic
Dysfunctional - Rationalist

Associated Animal
None

Societal Association
None

Sacramental Association
Ordination

Associated Sense
Sixth sense

Foods
None

Incense/Oils
Hyacinth, Violet, Rose geranium

Crystals
Amethyst, Purple apatite, Azurite, Calcite, Sapphire, Fluorite, Lapis lazuli

ARCHETYPES: THIRD EYE CHAKRA

The story of how my first book came into being illustrates perfectly the functional and dysfunctional archetypes of the Third Eye (Sixth) Chakra. An opportunity came up to write the book *(The Book of Crystal Healing)*, and I knew immediately that I was destined to do it, yet the two sides of my brain wrestled for supremacy before I took action. The left, logical, hemisphere "told" me that this was a strange and unusual subject and that perhaps it was not for me. But my right, creative, side simply trusted that writing this book was the way forward. It was as if I was being given a glimpse into the future. The book was going to be written by me, it was going to be a major success and eventually lead me into an area in which I could grow. Had I allowed my intellect to override my intuition I would never have directed my career on to a path that is now offering me both material and spiritual satisfaction and success. Yet how common it is for us to give way to the Rationalist inside all of us? This dysfunctional archetype allows the left brain dominance, usually because of the fear and insecurity we feel at dismantling the safe world in which we have become cocooned and constricted. In reality, Rationalists are not simply people who take a "scientific" view of everything. This group also embraces controllers and perfectionists - those who cannot accept the human failings of others and are similarly hard on themselves.

The functional archetype of this chakra is the Psychic, which doesn't just refer to those people who use their powers in a professional sense, but anyone who trusts that the answers to life's challenges lie within themselves. Having been awakened to the need to listen by developing the Throat (Fifth) Chakra, Psychics now listen to their inner Self. They recognize that the wisdom of the Third Eye Chakra is like a whisper that cannot be heard unless the cacophony of everyday life is stilled. Hence they recognize the need for meditation and contemplation in order for their creativity and intuition to shine through.

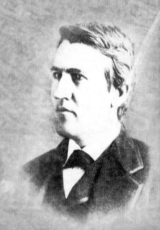

FRUITS OF THE IMAGINATION

Many scientists get stuck in the rut of rationalizing, intellectualizing, and theorizing. Yet the truly great scientists and inventors such as Albert Einstein and Thomas Edison freely acknowledged that their discoveries came from the imagination rather than logic. Many of Einstein's theories came from daydreams, including one where he imagined riding on a sunbeam and concluded that the Universe is both finite and curved.

THE PSYCHIC

Having honed their skills, Psychics often become exceptional artists, healers, and therapists. They know the difference between theory and practice - that the truly gifted individual is one who doesn't just "live by the book" but trusts their instincts to supply them with unique and telling insights.

THE RATIONALIST

Having chosen not to trust their feelings, insights, and inner wisdom - perhaps because these aspects of themselves were ridiculed in childhood - Rationalists force themselves to abide by a set of rules that becomes increasingly limiting and isolationist.

Experiment with the meditation, daily questions, and affirmations on pages 116-17 in order to let your Rationalist go and to nurture your Psychic's instincts.

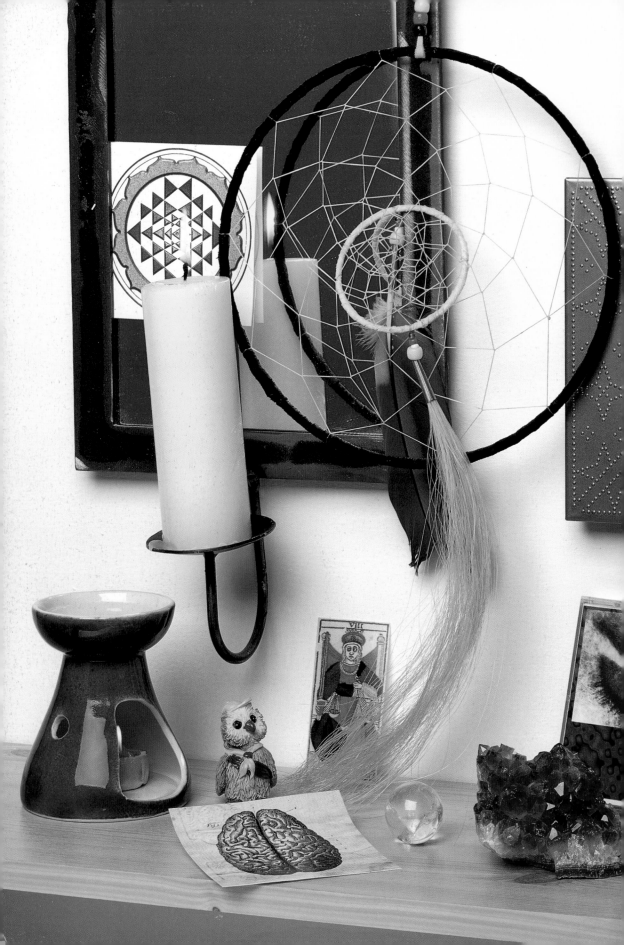

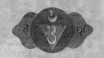

ALTAR:
THIRD EYE CHAKRA

James had always prided himself on his intellectual capabilities. He ran a small company and while an accomplished businessperson he found it difficult to attract the right employees. Often he would get a "gut feeling" about someone, but would ignore it - preferring to base his decision on paper qualifications. He would then find that his feelings about that person turned out to be more accurate than any "scientific" approach. Failing to tap into his intuition also meant that he sometimes got involved in unsuccessful business dealings. James struggled with learning to trust his "inner guide". His partner, recognizing that James' logical approach to human relations was not serving him, suggested they prepare an altar:

▽ An ornate mirror with in-built candle holder, representing light
▽ Oil burner containing Rose geranium
▽ Tarot card depicting Justice
▽ Small Quartz crystal ball
▽ Tapes of visualization exercises to enhance intuition
▽ Piece of Amethyst, said to encourage visionary abilities
▽ The Third Eye Chakra symbol
▽ Indigo-coloured mandala
▽ A dream-catcher
▽ Pottery owl, for wisdom
▽ Favourite lamp
▽ Picture of the brain, showing left and right hemispheres and the aptitudes ascribed to each

This altar is James' attempt to work on the Third Eye Chakra. It is a case study, for inspiration. Choose objects which have personal significance for you.

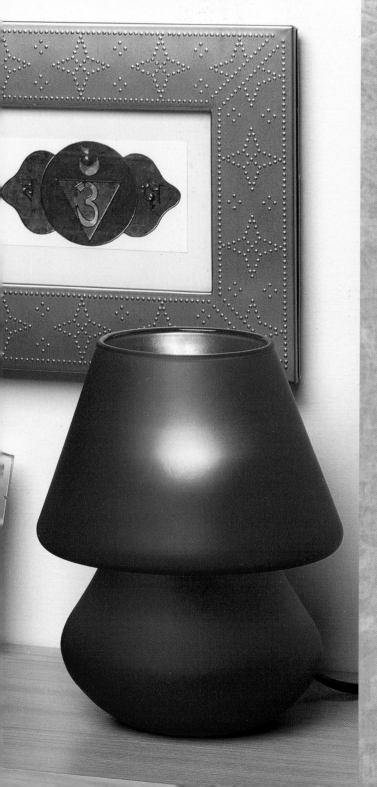

EXERCISE: THIRD EYE CHAKRA

Developing your ability to visualize colour offers
you another tool with which to access the
messages and creativity of the Third Eye. Adopt a
relaxed, comfortable position. Rest your gaze on
the empty mandala (see facing page - take a black
and white photocopy, which will look "empty") -
or any other similarly abstract, colourless drawing
that appeals to you.

1. Imagine a beam of white light, which comprises
all the colours of the rainbow, shining down through
the Crown of your head into the sushumna (see
p.17). Allow your imagination to extract each of the
rainbow colours in turn from this white light, in
order to project them in your mind's eye on to the
blank mandala.

2. First "pull down" the red of the Root (1st)
Chakra and fill all the white spaces of the mandala with red. Then focus your attention back
on the beam of white light and pull down the
orange hue. Let your imagination wash the
mandala with the colour orange.

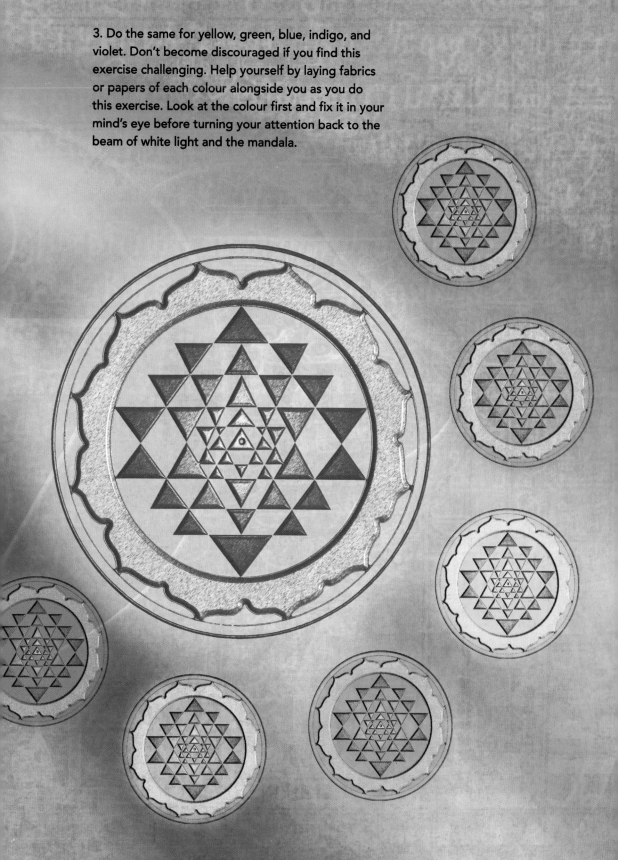

3. Do the same for yellow, green, blue, indigo, and violet. Don't become discouraged if you find this exercise challenging. Help yourself by laying fabrics or papers of each colour alongside you as you do this exercise. Look at the colour first and fix it in your mind's eye before turning your attention back to the beam of white light and the mandala.

KEY CRYSTALS: THIRD EYE CHAKRA

Crystals that enhance intuition and psychic abilities include those that resonate to bluish-purple indigo. Some crystals (e.g. Amethyst) can be used on more than one chakra. This is perfectly acceptable; the relevance will be influenced both by the variation in shade and the power of your intention. (See also pp.26-7 for information on Crystal Healing.)

CALCITE

A crystal that can be found in a wide range of colours, depending on what other minerals were in contact during formation. It can be used on various chakras, but clear Calcite helps to amplify the energies of the Third Eye, bringing about a greater spiritual appreciation of the intuitive side.

PURPLE FLUORITE

Fluorite occurs in many forms and colours and has been known as the "stone of discernment", said to bring together rationality and intuition. Used on the Third Eye Chakra it facilitates the opening of an infinite range of mental avenues, increases the ability to concentrate and strips away false illusions. Purple fluorite assists in the ability to articulate information attained psychically.

AZURITE

Used on the Third Eye Chakra, this lustrous crystal awakens the development of psychic abilities and helps promote the desire to act on intuitive information. It is a beneficial stone for stimulating a blocked or under-utilized Third Eye. The Mayans used this crystal to facilitate the transfer of inner wisdom and knowledge to normal thought

AMETHYST

Ranging in colour from deep purple to pale lavender, Amethyst is the "stone of meditation" and is equally useful for the Third Eye and the Crown Chakra. It has a beneficial, protective, energy and imparts a calming influence if you are swept away by intellectual and emotional turmoil. (See also pp.128-9.)

JAMES (see also pp.110-11)

Because of his sceptical, "left brain", approach to crystal healing, James was reluctant to try a full layout, but was persuaded to use a small piece of Amethyst at the Third Eye Chakra to help him medi- tate. He agreed to set aside two half-hour periods every day in which he would lie down and relax, place the Amethyst on his brow and listen to tapes varying from nature sounds to guided visualizations. The lat- ter were specially written to usher in an acceptance of the intuitive self. In addition, James was given several affirmations to repeat while gazing at a large bed of Amethyst placed on his desk. These included the sug- gestion of freeing his mind from its logical constraints and to trust his Higher Self to provide the answers to any questions.

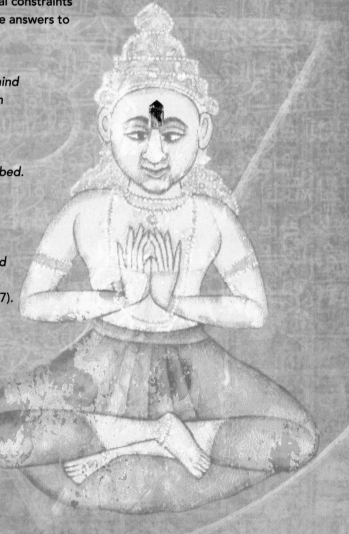

Approach crystal healing with an open mind and take the time to choose and position crystals with your needs and wishes uppermost.

▽ *Choose a warm, comfortable place.*
▽ *Ensure you are not going to be disturbed.*
▽ *Play gentle music or nature sounds.*
▽ *Burn incense or scented candles.*
▽ *Wear loose clothes.*
▽ *Go to the bathroom first.*
▽ *Have a glass of water to rehydrate and ground you afterwards.*
▽ *Cleanse and tune the crystals (see p.27).*

MEDITATION: THIRD EYE CHAKRA

Before you start
Choose a leisurely and relaxed time to meditate.
▽ Sit or lie before your altar (see pp.110-11). Let the colours, symbols, and associations inspire you.
▽ Create atmosphere with oils, candles, or incense.
▽ Tape the words if you like. Dots indicate a pause.

1. Assume a comfortable position and breathe slowly and deeply through your nose.

2. Tense each set of muscles in turn, from feet and ankles to neck and head ...
and as they relax feel yourself sink heavily into the floor or chair ...

3. In your mind's eye become aware of the Third Eye Chakra, positioned between your eyebrows, as if it were a physical entity ...

4. Focus on the twin white wings of the Ajna symbol
on either side of a circle (see p.106) ...
See a golden triangle within that circle, pointing downward toward the earth ...
connecting your Higher Consciousness with your physical entity ...

5. Now flood that symbol with the colour indigo so that it
bathes your forehead with violet-blue ...
violet washing down from the Crown Chakra at the top of your head ...
and blue moving up from the Throat Chakra at the base of your neck ...

6. Your Third Eye Chakra is a beautiful lotus flower ...
feel its roots go deep within your forehead, connecting with the
sushumna, the central column linking the stems of each chakra ...

7. Feel the energy of the Third Eye vortex as it spins
effortlessly between your physical eyes ...
sense the pulsation of chakra energy ... be aware of any other sensations -
smell the fragrance of the Third Eye Chakra lotus ...

8. The Third Eye is as real as your two physical eyes ...
it is there to offer you insight, clairvoyance, truths to
the questions of the universe ...
nurture it as carefully as you would your physical eyes ... exercise it daily ...
let your intuition guide you daily, leading you to a more fulfilling, joyous life.

DAILY QUESTIONS

▽ How much silence is there in your life for the whispers of intuition to be heard? Spend time in silence. Focus on something beautiful and be still and silent.

▽ When did you last act on intuition? Go with any compelling thoughts, without rationalization. Be alert to coincidences and experiences that may contain messages.

▽ Do you truly see what is around you? Exercise your physical perception by being alert to details, such as shapes and colours.

▽ Do you look outside yourself for answers? List personal queries, such as why a certain person has come into your life. Note insights in the form of images, colours, words, or phrases.

AFFIRMATIONS

▽ I recognize the need for silence and stillness in my life.

▽ The answers to all my questions lie within me.

▽ I trust my inner self to guide and protect me.

▽ I trust my feelings.

▽ I have nothing to prove. I am the Divine Plan manifesting itself.

▽ I am full of wisdom.

▽ I trust that my imagination will create a world of happiness and security for me.

▽ Imagination is the life-blood of my creativity.

▽ I choose to accept myself and others exactly as we are.

▽ Making mistakes enables me to learn, grow, and develop.

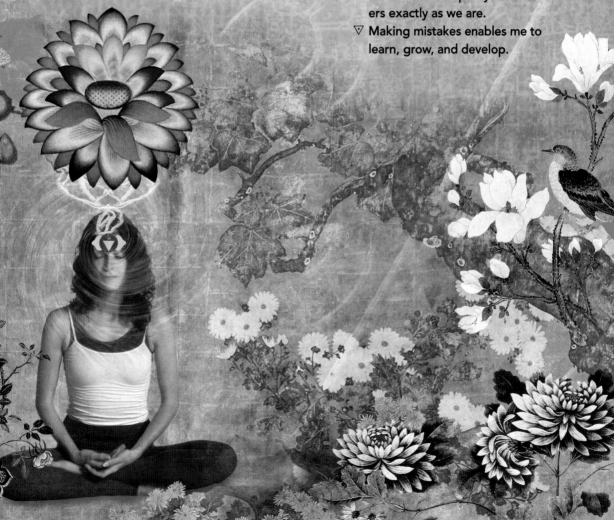

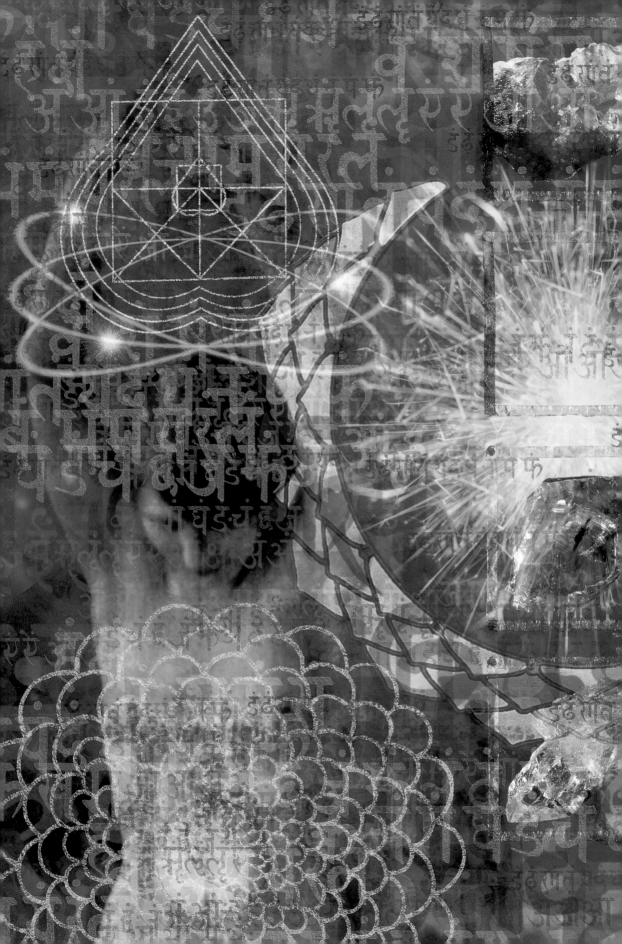

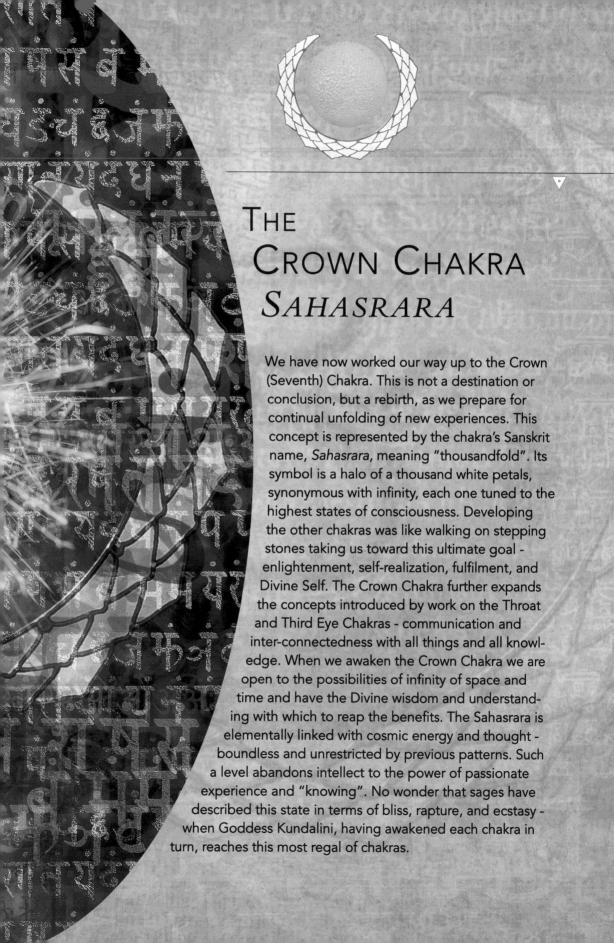

THE
CROWN CHAKRA
SAHASRARA

We have now worked our way up to the Crown (Seventh) Chakra. This is not a destination or conclusion, but a rebirth, as we prepare for continual unfolding of new experiences. This concept is represented by the chakra's Sanskrit name, *Sahasrara*, meaning "thousandfold". Its symbol is a halo of a thousand white petals, synonymous with infinity, each one tuned to the highest states of consciousness. Developing the other chakras was like walking on stepping stones taking us toward this ultimate goal - enlightenment, self-realization, fulfilment, and Divine Self. The Crown Chakra further expands the concepts introduced by work on the Throat and Third Eye Chakras - communication and inter-connectedness with all things and all knowledge. When we awaken the Crown Chakra we are open to the possibilities of infinity of space and time and have the Divine wisdom and understanding with which to reap the benefits. The Sahasrara is elementally linked with cosmic energy and thought - boundless and unrestricted by previous patterns. Such a level abandons intellect to the power of passionate experience and "knowing". No wonder that sages have described this state in terms of bliss, rapture, and ecstasy - when Goddess Kundalini, having awakened each chakra in turn, reaches this most regal of chakras.

CROWN CHAKRA CORRESPONDENCES

This chart for the Crown (Seventh) Chakra identifies all the associations and symbolisms linked with this particular chakra. As such it provides a "ready reference" of inspirations to use when you carry out practical exercises such as assembling your altar arrangements (see pp.124-5) or choosing appropriate stones for crystal work (pp.128-9). This chart will also help you with the various images you will need when composing your own meditations and visualizations. Incorporate as many of these symbols and themes as you feel is appropriate to your needs.

By reacquainting yourself regularly with this chakra chart as a prelude to the section on the Crown Chakra, you will help to keep your mind focused on related issues, including the reprogramming of dysfunctional patterns of thought and behaviour.

Our journey through the chakras has led us to a new horizon and from this spiritual perspective has expanded our consciousnesses, so that we live more fulfilled, joyous, and healthy lives.

CHAKRA CHARACTERISTICS

See which of the following characteristics of excessive ("too open"), deficient ("blocked"), and balanced chakra energy you can relate to - and then determine (should you choose) to take the necessary action, using the tools and techniques outlined in this chapter.

Too open (chakra spins too fast) - psychotic or manic depressive, confused sexual expression, frustrated, sense of unrealized power
Blocked (chakra spins sluggishly or not at all) - constantly exhausted, can't make decisions, no sense of "belonging"
Balanced (chakra maintains equilibrium and spins at correct vibrational speed) - magnetic personality, achieves "miracles" in life, transcendent, at peace with self

THE CROWN CHAKRA

Sanskrit Name
Sahasrara

Meaning
Thousandfold

Location
Top/crown of head

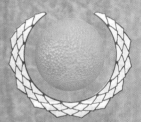

Symbol
The 1000-petalled lotus flower

Associated Colours
Violet, gold, white

Element
Thought, cosmic energy

Ruling Planet
Uranus

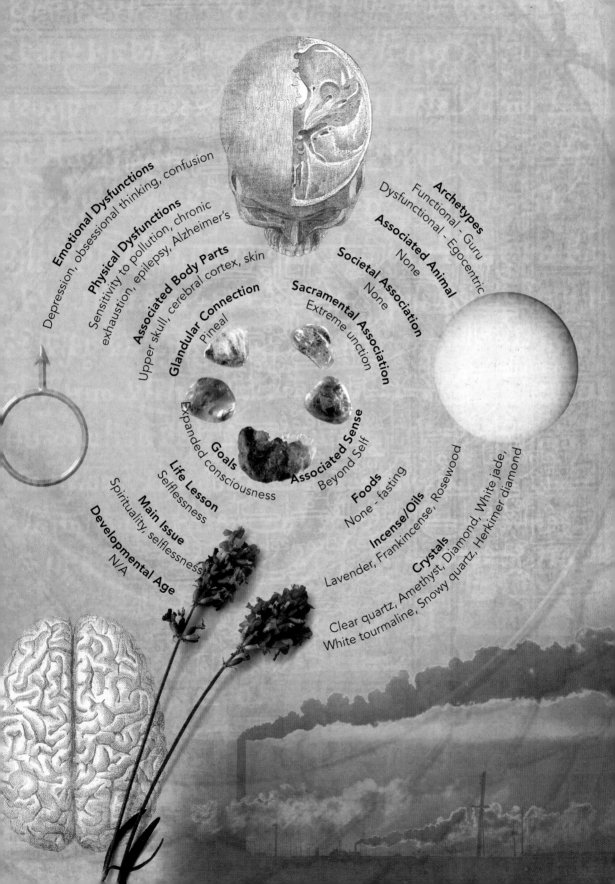

Emotional Dysfunctions
Depression, obsessional thinking, confusion

Physical Dysfunctions
Sensitivity to pollution, chronic exhaustion, epilepsy, Alzheimer's

Associated Body Parts
Upper skull, cerebral cortex, skin

Glandular Connection
Pineal

Goals
Expanded consciousness

Life Lesson
Selflessness

Main Issue
Spirituality, selflessness

Developmental Age
N/A

Archetypes
Functional - Guru
Dysfunctional - Egocentric

Associated Animal
None

Societal Association
None

Sacramental Association
Extreme unction

Associated Sense
Beyond Self

Foods
None - fasting

Incense/Oils
Lavender, Frankincense, Rosewood

Crystals
Clear quartz, Amethyst, Diamond, White jade, White tourmaline, Snowy quartz, Herkimer diamond

ARCHETYPES: CROWN CHAKRA

Success and spirituality are not mutually exclusive. However, when the former is sought at the expense of the latter the resulting imbalanced state illustrates the difference between the positive and negative archetypes of the Crown (Seventh) Chakra - the Guru and the Egocentric.

A common expression of Egocentric is "I make my own luck". Because of their total focus on the material world and the illusion of their control over it, Egocentrics have no awareness of, nor relationship with, the Divine. These control-junkies regard themselves as wholly responsible for all the benefits they accrue in life. Indeed, their psychological well-being largely depends on material success, since Egocentrics identify themselves solely in terms of what they do, not who they are. The problem is that they are so busy focusing on their destination that they neglect to enjoy the journey and their tendency to workaholism often leaves them lonely and unfulfilled at the deepest level.

The Egocentric world view is mechanistic in that they have no time for anything that cannot be explained logically. Hence they fail to draw benefit from all that is mysterious and inexplicable in life. It is sometimes only late in life, when the trappings of success - particularly status at work - have been stripped from them through retirement or redundancy (or their health suffers because of their relentless "good living" lifestyle), that Egocentrics are forced to confront their spiritual bankruptcy.

The title Guru is no longer only applicable to a mystic sitting on a mountain top meditating life away. I believe that this state is equally achievable by those whose worldly success is as great as that of the Egocentric. However, Gurus take an expansive view of their world situation. They may focus on specific, attainable, goals, but know that there are infinite possibilities - more than the human mind alone can fathom - through which those goals might be realized. Therefore they are open to, and embrace, the unexpected, the serendipitous, the coincidental. Unlike the arrogant, self-centred Egocentric, Gurus accept how little they know and trust that their connection to their Higher Self will always provide the right answer or pathway. These individu-

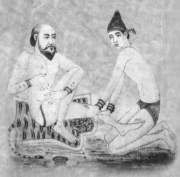

THE EGOCENTRIC CRISIS

A crisis point in mid-life occurs when a deep longing for meaning and purpose fails to be assuaged by material success. The cry "Is that it?", "Is this all my life is about?" is common for Egocentrics. Traumatic experiences may find them floundering. Why does sheer willpower no longer serve? It is only then that the Egocentric can learn the lesson which the Guru has already long embraced - the surrender to Divine Will or "a detachment from outcomes".

i4 pg

als radiate an inner calm that comes from a total acceptance of who - not what - they truly are. These are not human beings trying to be spiritual, but spiritual beings learning vital emotional lessons through temporarily wearing the cloak of humanity.

THE GURU

This archetype, in many respects, holds the key to living successfully on this earth, in the acceptance of personal limitations and the awareness that all things are possible.

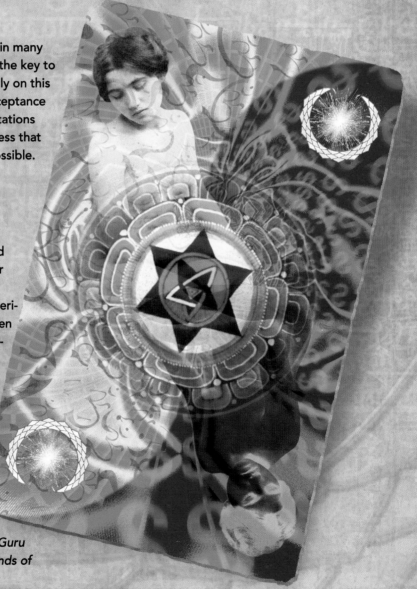

THE EGOCENTRIC

Self-determination and tight control over their own lives make Egocentrics value materialism, only to find, when this is no longer meaningful, that they lack the inner resources to get more from life.

The meditation, daily questions, and affirmations on pages 130-1 will help you achieve connection with your Guru and release the demands of the Egocentric.

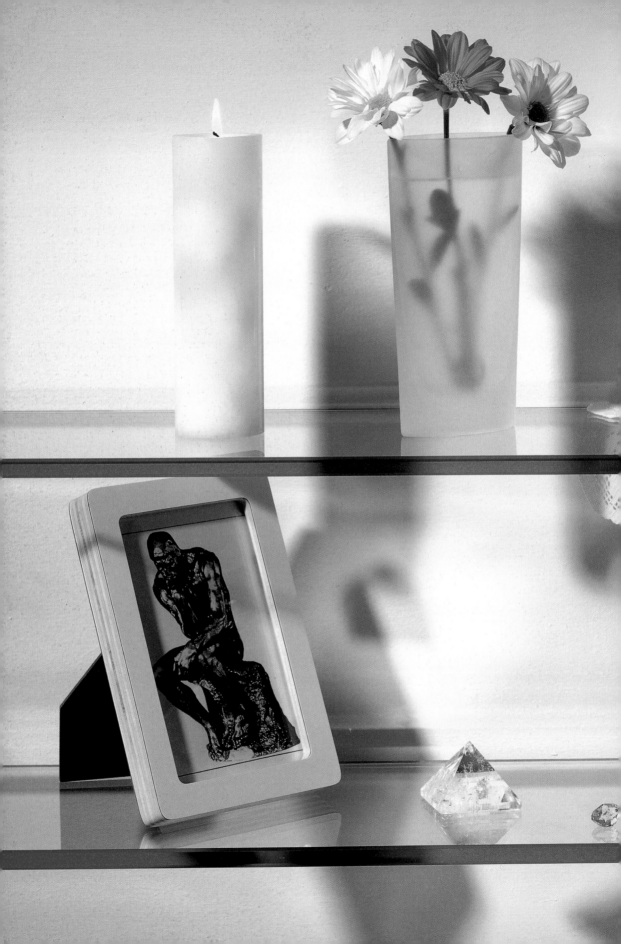

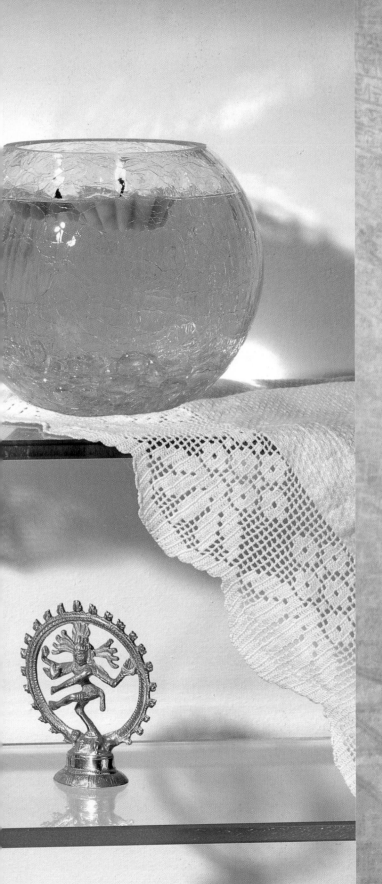

ALTAR: CROWN CHAKRA

After many successful years' running her own consultancy, Jenny realized that the material possessions she once craved no longer satisfied her. She had shocked her friends by announcing she was going to simplify her life, sell her city home, and work freelance from her favourite country area - renowned for its natural beauty and spiritual connections. Jenny was determined to demonstrate that it is possible to be "spiritual" while maintaining a practical, earthly existence. She recognized that, while it is nice to own beautiful objects, possessions are only "things"; not the sum total of one's self. One of the first things Jenny did in her new home was create an altar to represent giving up her previously held material values. Her altar is beautiful but sparse:

▽ Frosted glass vase containing fresh white and violet flowers
▽ Delicate white altar cloth, a gift from her dearest friend
▽ Herkimer diamond, believed to enhance spiritual qualities
▽ Small gold-coloured model of the Hindu God, Shiva
▽ Clear glass bowl of water containing glass pebbles and petalled floating candles, representing a thousand-petalled lotus
▽ Single white candle
▽ Clear quartz pyramid
▽ Picture of Rodin's *The Thinker*, for the element of thought

This altar is Jenny's attempt to work on the Crown Chakra. It is a case study, for inspiration. Choose objects which have personal significance for you.

Exercise: Crown Chakra

Provided you don't have a heart condition, high blood pressure, or eye problems - you can achieve a headstand with a little patience and practice. Inverting the body counters the negative effects of gravity. Benefits include improved circulation, prevention and alleviation of back problems, better memory and concentration, and a different experience of time and space. Take time to ensure that your hands and elbows are in the correct position before attempting to lift your feet off the floor. Breathing may seem difficult at first, inhalation tends to be deeper in the inverted state.

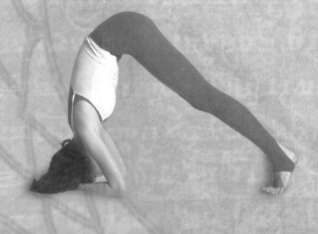

1. Kneel on a soft mat and rest your forearms on top of each other, holding the opposite elbow with each hand. Keeping your elbows in this position, release your hands and place them in front of you, fingers intertwined. Lower your head to rest on the floor, with your clasped hands holding the back of it. Keep your elbows in position throughout the sequence. Straighten your knees and raise your hips so that your body forms a triangle with the floor.

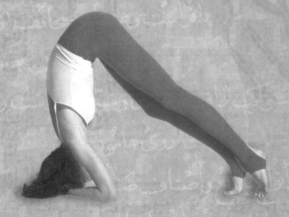

2. Keeping your knees straight and your neck directly in line with your spine, walk slowly toward your head as far as you can.

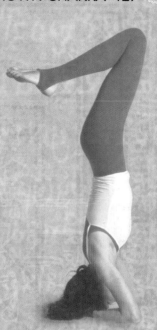

3. Bend your knees toward your chest and lift your feet off the floor, pausing to ensure your hips are tilted slightly backward.

4. Still with bent knees, lift your legs into the air by using your abdominal muscles.

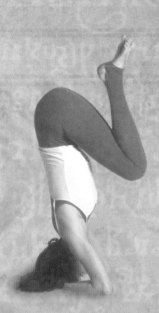

5. When you feel secure, slowly stretch your legs toward the ceiling, resting your body's weight on your forearms. Gradually build up the length of time you remain in the headstand, particularly if you are unused to it. When completed, reverse the sequence to come down.

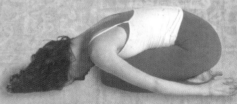

6. Give your body time to normalize itself after a headstand. Do this by kneeling down, resting your buttocks on your feet with toes pointing outward. Rest your forehead on the floor and relax your arms in a backward position so that your upturned palms rest alongside your feet. Stay in this position for at least six deep nasal breaths.

KEY CRYSTALS: CROWN CHAKRA

The clarity of perception and self-understanding achieved when the Crown Chakra functions properly, corresponds with the transparency of many crystals used for the Crown. Clear and colourless Quartz crystals are particularly useful, since all the rainbow colours combined in equal proportion produce white light. (See also pp.26-7 for information on Crystal Healing.)

CLEAR QUARTZ
A wonderful "all purpose" crystal for meditation or healing which can amplify, focus, and transform energy, bringing balance and harmony to any chakra. It is believed to help encourage altered states of consciousness and assist movement of Kundalini energy to bring about a realization of spiritual power.

HERKIMER DIAMOND
A unique form of quartz commonly found as short, double-terminated crystals. These diamonds help bring about a harmony of energy throughout the body, prompting self-acceptance and a desire to "be" rather than "do". Said to be an excellent anti-depressant if worn in a pocket.

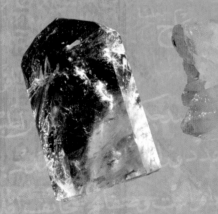

AMETHYST
This crystal is said to open and activate the Crown Chakra, balance the energies of the physical, emotional, and mental bodies and help facilitate a sense of spirituality and contentment. An excellent meditation stone, it assists the mind in surrendering to the Higher Self. Its message is: "Let go and trust".

DIAMOND
The Italian for diamond, *amante de Dio*, means "lover of God" and this most precious crystal is said to stimulate far sightedness and spirituality. The Diamond is the symbol of perfection, enabling us to move toward our highest spiritual potential. Its brilliance is believed to keep negativity at bay.

JENNY (see also pp.124-5)

A full body layout was used to help Jenny achieve altered states of consciousness in which to connect with her Higher Self. She placed the following crystals on each chakra to balance her whole system:

▽ **Smoky quartz** - at the Root Chakra (see pp.44-5);
▽ **Golden topaz** - at the Sacral Chakra (see pp.58-9);
▽ **Malachite** - at the Solar Plexus Chakra (see pp.72-3);
▽ **Rose quartz** - at the Heart Chakra (see pp.86-7);
▽ **Aquamarine and Celestite** - at the Throat Chakra (see pp.100-1);
▽ **Amethyst** - at the Third Eye Chakra (see pp.114-15);
▽ **Single-terminated Clear quartz** - pointing upward at the Crown Chakra.

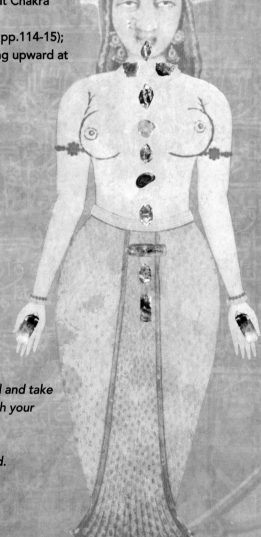

Additionally, Jenny held single-terminated Clear quartz crystals in her hands and placed them at the base of her feet, with the pointed ends toward her body to circulate healing energy. Herkimer diamonds were positioned between each of the chakras to help provide a clear passage for the energy to flow between them.

Approach crystal healing with an open mind and take the time to choose and position crystals with your needs and wishes uppermost.

▽ *Choose a warm, comfortable place.*
▽ *Ensure you are not going to be disturbed.*
▽ *Play gentle music or nature sounds.*
▽ *Burn incense or scented candles.*
▽ *Wear loose clothes.*
▽ *Go to the bathroom first.*
▽ *Have a glass of water to rehydrate and ground you afterwards.*
▽ *Cleanse and tune the crystals (see p.27).*

MEDITATION: CROWN CHAKRA

Before you start
Choose a leisurely and relaxed time to meditate.
▽ Sit or lie before your altar (see pp.124-5). Let the colours, symbols, and associations inspire you.
▽ Create atmosphere with oils, candles, or incense.
▽ Tape the words if you like. Dots indicate a pause.

1. As you sit or lie in your warm, silent, safe place, imagine a cap of a thousand white petals hugging the crown of your head.

2. Through the centre, where the petals meet, is an opening through which pours a golden/white/violet (choose) light ... This is your link with the Divine Source ... your connection with everything that ever was, is, or will be ...

3. Allow this light to pour in throughout your body ... nurturing every cell, every fibre of your being ... with pure consciousness ...

4. A consciousness that transcends normal thought and the ordinary senses ... A consciousness taking you beyond space and time into a state of deeper awareness ...

5. This is your link with an unlimited realm of understanding, of knowing ...

6. The ability to trust that everything in your life is unfolding exactly as it should, for your highest good ... Feel the power of this connection as the light bathes your body internally and externally with its Divine Radiance ...

7. You are becoming enlightened ... the process of unlocking the mental blocks that have chained you to mundane realities in the past ...

8. Now you allow your mind to soar above its earthly shackles and detach itself from the limitations of your mortal mind ...

9. By doing so you are attaching yourself to your Higher Self ... to new experiences ... new beginnings ... a new awakening.

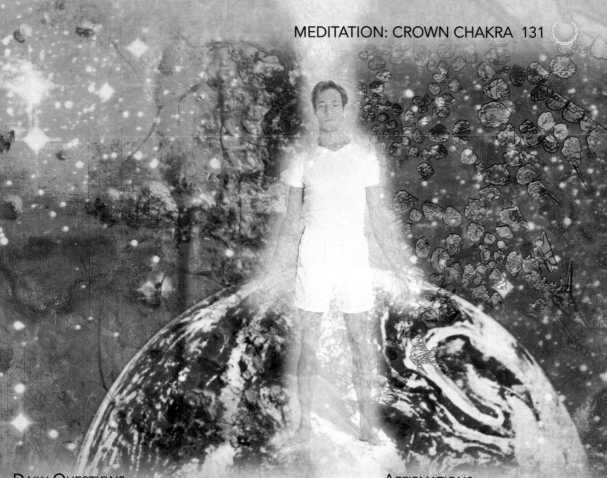

DAILY QUESTIONS

▽ Do you retread familiar thought and behaviour patterns? Move into uncharted territory, available when you explore your Crown Chakra.

▽ Does your personal identification begin and end with job or economic status? List words describing the essential you. Add to the list daily.

▽ Can you reserve time for daily meditation? This is the key to achieving enlightenment.

▽ Do you believe that you too can achieve mystical states of consciousness? Read about ordinary people whose lives have been transformed by a more enlightened lifestyle.

▽ Are you in control of your destiny? Think back to when something wonderful happened. Did you control that event? Be open to coincidences that add magic to your life.

▽ Is there an issue in your life which you are battling to control through sheer willpower? Practice letting go of your desired outcome. Take a deep breath and tell yourself, "I trust that the outcome will be for my highest good, no matter what it may be." Then let go.

AFFIRMATIONS

▽ I tune into the union with my Higher Power.

▽ I am starting to accept myself as I am, with love and gratitude.

▽ I cease to limit myself intellectually and in my creativity and connect my spirit to the Source of all knowledge.

▽ I am a unique, radiant, loving being.

▽ I choose to live my life from a place of love and contentment.

▽ I choose to transform my life and become free.

▽ I release all limited thoughts and lift myself up to ever higher levels of awareness.

▽ I am who I am and glory in that.

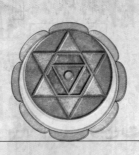

INTEGRATED APPROACHES

Chakra balancing is usually combined with other alternative therapies, since holistic approaches require an understanding of the chakras for healing the physical, emotional, and spiritual aspects of the self. Increasingly, practitioners across a broad range of disciplines have studied how chi energy, transmitted through the chakras, has profound impacts on well-being. This could be what marks the difference between a good therapist, extensively trained, with widespread experience, and a true healer; someone whose own balanced chakra energy offers an added dimension to their work with others. While it is not possible to cover every area in which knowledge of the chakras enhances a particular approach, here are four popular disciplines making extensive use of the system:

AROMATHERAPY

Aromatherapy is both an art and a science, where the essential oils of plants and flowers are used to heal, beautify, and boost emotional and spiritual well-being. At a chemical level, essential oils comprise various physical components, which, applied to the skin, enter the bloodstream and are carried around the body. However, there is another view that says these essences can assist in vibrational healing, since they contain the Universal Life Force energy, or "soul", of the plant, and that it is this which interacts with our own chi energy to stimulate, subdue, or balance the chakras. Aromatherapists who integrate an understanding of the chakras into

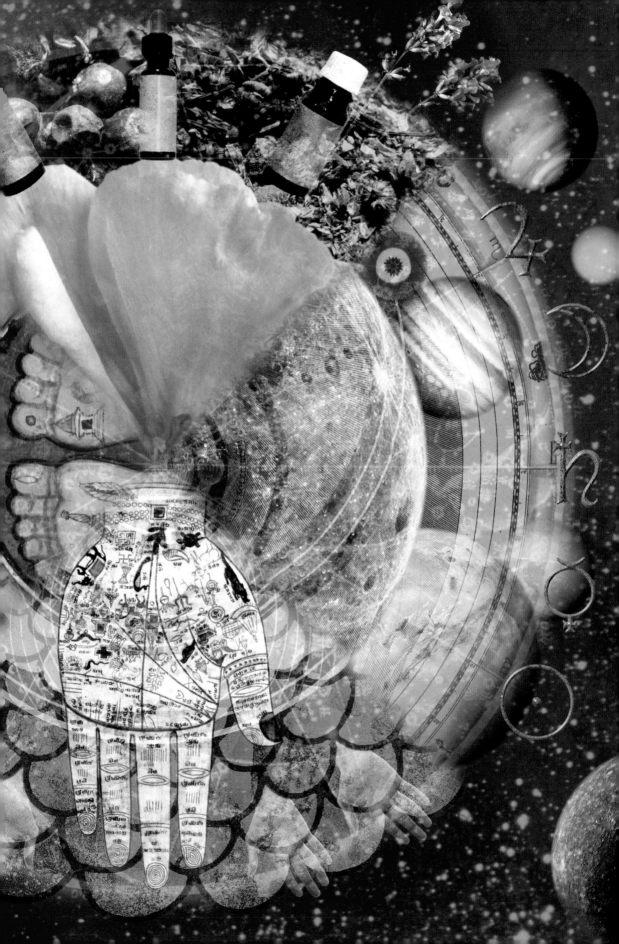

their work to achieve a balance of the sevenfold system often look for a link between the colour of the oil or flower. For example, essential oils for the Root (First) Chakra, relating to grounding and centring, include brown or reddish base notes such as Myrrh, Vetivert, and Cedarwood. No two experts agree on which oils work best on which chakra, since oils can influence individuals differently, depending on whether they require energizing, calming, or balancing. As with all intuitive work, harmony in the body and mind is best restored by following personal preferences. Therefore a good aromatherapist will always ask you to smell and agree on the oils s/he has chosen first.

REIKI

Reiki is another important form of "energy medicine", where practitioners, having been "attuned" to Reiki energy in special ceremonies (given by a Reiki Master), become "channels" of Universal Life Force, or Reiki, energy. They transmit energy by placing their hands on specific areas, including the chakras, using special hand positions. The resulting balancing of energies can work on a physical, mental, emotional, or spiritual level, depending upon the receiver's needs. The physical manifestation of the healing energy of a Reiki practitioner is the warmth, or "heat", radiating from the hands. Many people have explored Reiki simply for the deeply relaxing experience it offers. Others say that they benefit from its regular energy "re-tuning". Reiki is also said to help relieve pain, and while no claims are made that it can "cure" chronic conditions, many sufferers have found that quality of life is enhanced by the physical and psychological relief of balanced energies.

REFLEXOLOGY

The ancient art of applying pressure to parts of the foot to affect a related area or organ was first practised by early Eastern healers thousands of years ago. However, it was not until 1913 that ear, nose, and throat consultant, Dr William Fitzgerald, introduced Zone Therapy, now called Reflexology, to the West. Reflexologists regard the feet as mirroring the body, with the toes representing the head and brains, down to the heels, which correspond to the pelvic area. Where there are parts of the body on both the left and the right side (such as the kidneys), the reflexologist will work on the corresponding parts of both feet. In some cases, as with the heart, s/he will only work on the left foot. In the same way that a reflexologist will apply gentle pressure to all parts of the feet, noting discomfort, indicating a blockage in the corresponding part of the body, some practitioners work specifically on the chakras to help with a particular dysfunction or emotional issue. This is done by focusing on the vital energy pathways, or "meridians", which are related to the glands and organs associated with each chakra. While reflexology is commonly thought of as a means of treating physical illness, a therapist with knowledge of the chakra system can extend their expertise to the mental and emotional self.

ASTROLOGY

As long ago as 5 BC astrologer-priests in Mesopotamia linked the steps taken by the soul in its metaphysical journey toward enlightenment to planetary archetypes. Today, astrologers who consider their science to be another tool for personal understanding and transformation also use the planets and signs of the zodiac to illustrate the lessons and challenges we seek to learn during each incarnation. The planets illustrate different hierarchies of meaning and symbolize the experiences, characteristics, and life events we encounter during this voyage into the different levels of consciousness. It is believed that being born at a certain time and a particular set of planetary positions is a personal chart of the karmic lessons we have "chosen" to undertake in this lifetime. The following is a brief explanation of each of the planetary and chakra associations:

Root (First) Chakra/Saturn

Saturn represents the earthly baggage that prevents us moving toward our Higher Self; its position in our birth chart indicates where we place unnecessary limitations on ourselves, often imposed by society, culture, and family. Saturn also represents ego, fears, doubts, rules, and the need to control on which we base our security but which inevitably weigh us down and imprison us.

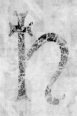

Sacral (Second) Chakra/Pluto

The mythological god of the underworld, Pluto rules the sex organs and represents instinctual and primitive urges - such as the drive for sex and all things hidden and secretive. Death and sex have traditionally been linked in mythology, poetry, and stories such as Bram Stoker's Dracula.

Solar Plexus (Third) Chakra/Sun and Mars

This chakra's associations of personal power as a prime source of energy can be related to the Sun, with which it has direct symbolisms and colour connection. The secondary planetary connection, Mars, is a proactive planet, prompting action and a bold spirit which fits with the Solar Plexus goals of endurance and sense of purpose.

Heart (Fourth) Chakra/Venus

Mythological Venus, the Greek Goddess Aphrodite, is traditionally associated with love. Like the Heart Chakra, which bridges the lower and higher chakras, Venus represents the dual aspect of earthly desire and passion and the Divine, more ephemeral, nature of love.

Throat (Fifth) Chakra/Mercury

Mercury, or Hermes, is the mythological messenger of the gods whose staff was the caduceus, with which the entire chakra system is symbolized. Mercury is the planet of communication and represents our ability to articulate our thoughts but also to interpret accurately what we hear from others.

Third Eye (Sixth) Chakra/Neptune and Jupiter

Neptune is considered to be the planetary archetype that opens the doors to our perception and allows us to experience the ecstasy of spirit through creativity. Its challenge in a chart is to accept what we pick up through intuition without needing to rationalize it, and hence reject things in favour of more tangible materialism. Jupiter, was, prior to the discovery of Neptune, said to be connected with telepathic thought.

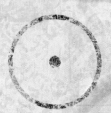
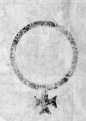
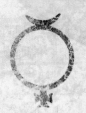
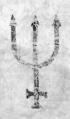

Crown (Seventh) Chakra/Uranus

Uranus is the consciousness-raising planet, affording us spiritual mastery. It offers us the ability to rise above the material plane and to see the "bigger picture". Its spirituality is one of detachment - of freeing ourselves from needing to know outcomes, of trusting that life offers more than we can possibly imagine.

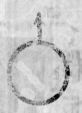

EPILOGUE

I hope that this book has inspired you to consider ways in which you can bring your chakras into balance within your daily life. The wide variety of inspirations offered take into account that you are a unique individual and will therefore be excited by something quite different from your neighbour. Always honour that individuality and amend the suggestions offered according to your intuitive needs.

If you have already set up an altar, tried out some of the physical exercises, or been prompted to write a daily journal exploring the psycho-emotional issues around certain chakra blockages, you might like to reflect on how different you feel since you first opened this book. What has changed in your life, both internally and externally? However, whatever stage you are at in your journey through the chakras, be assured that simply bringing the need for balance into your consciousness will move you inexorably toward that state. Taking action simply accelerates the process.

I have already said that knowledge is power. By getting to know yourself a little better, by applying the techniques offered in this book to your own life challenges, I sincerely wish you an increasingly powerful, satisfying, and enjoyable renaissance as a balanced and whole human being.

As Dolly Parton said: *"Find out who you are; then do it on purpose."*

GLOSSARY

Affirmation
A positive, personally inspiring phrase that acts as a powerful healing tool to counteract previous negative conditioning.

Altar
A focal point for meditation and contemplation, usually displaying a personal collection of meaningful possessions. Sometimes a ritual is involved to enhance the experience.

Archetype
A universal theme, or model, of human emotional development or rites of passage.

Aura
The "subtle" energy field surrounding the physical body, invisible to all but gifted individuals and through processes such as aura scans and Kirlian photography.

Block/blockage
A dysfunction in the chakra system inhibiting the smooth, even flow of subtle energy.

Chakras
An integrated system of metaphysical energy centres which affect physical, mental, emotional, and spiritual well-being.

Crystal
Solid material with ordered internal atomic structure of regularly repeating three-dimensional patterns.

Endocrine system
One of the body's major physical control systems that transmits hormones produced from a series of ductless glands throughout the physical body. The system corresponds broadly to the positions of the seven major chakras.

Grounding
The importance of maintaining connection to the Earth in order to be fully centred.

Higher Self
That part of ourselves from which, once tuned in, we can receive Divine Guidance.

Kundalini
Mythical serpent goddess said to rise through the chakras in the journey toward enlightenment.

Lingam
Hindu phallus, a symbol of Shiva.

Mandala
An abstract universal symbol, used as an aid to meditation and to achieve higher states of consciousness.

Meridian
A channel through which subtle energy flows in the body.

Subtle body/energy
That part of our Selves which resonates at vibrational levels, invisible to "normal" sight.

Sushumna
Energetic equivalent of the spine; the vertical column within which the major chakra system is located.

Universal Life Force
Inexplicable, natural source of life which plays a vital role in health and healing.

Yin and yang
According to Ancient Chinese philosopy, the two opposing but complementary forces at work in nature.

BIBLIOGRAPHY

Angelo, Jack, *Your Healing Power*, Piatkus Books, 1994

Breathnach, Sarah Ban, *Simple Abundance: A Daybook of Comfort and Joy*, Transworld, 1996

Brennan, Barbara Ann, *Hands of Light: A Guide to Healing Through The Human Energy Field*, Bantam, 1987

Dale, Cyndi, *New Chakra Healing*, Llewellyn Publications, 1997

Davis, Patricia, *Subtle Aromatherapy*, C.W. Daniel, 1991

Evans, John, *Mind, Body and Electromagnetism*, Element Books, 1986

Furlong, David, *The Complete Healer*, Piatkus Books, 1995

Gardner, Joy, *Color and Crystals: A Journey Through the Chakras*, The Crossing Press, 1988

Honervogt, Tanmaya, *Reiki: Healing and Harmony Through the Hands*, Gaia Books, 1998

Hodgson, Joan, *The Stars and the Chakras: The Astrology of Spiritual Unfoldment*, The White Eagle Publishing Trust, 1990

Hunt, Valerie V., *Infinite Mind: The Science of Human Vibrations*, Malibu Publishing Co., 1995

Judith, Anodea, *Wheels of Life: A User's Guide to the Chakra System*, Llewellyn Publications, 1996

Karagulla, Shafica MD and Van Gelder Kunz, Dora, *The Chakras and the Human Energy Fields*, The Theosophical Publishing House, 1989

Melody, *Love is in the Earth - A Kaleidoscope of Crystals*, Earth-Love Publishing House, 1995

Myss, Caroline, *Anatomy of the Spirit: The Seven Stages of Power & Healing*, Bantam Books, 1997

Ozaniec, Naomi, *Chakras for Beginners*, Hodder & Stoughton-Headway, 1994

Raphaell, Katrina, *Crystal Enlightenment, vols. I & II*, Aurora Press, 1985

Simpson, Liz, *The Book of Crystal Healing*, Gaia Books, 1997

The Sivananda Yoga Centre, *The Book of Yoga - The Complete Step-by-Step Guide*, Ebury Press, 1983

Wauters, Ambika, *Journey of Self Discovery: How to Work With the Energies of Chakras and Archetypes*, Piatkus Books, 1996

White, Ruth, *Working With Your Chakras*, Piatkus Books, 1993

RESOURCES

The College of Psychic Studies
16 Queensbury Place
London SW7 2EB
(offers a team of healers and intuitives who work with the chakras)

White Eagle Lodge
New Lands
Brewells Lane
Liss
Hants GU33 7HY
(offers healing courses and training, integrating their own method of chakra work)

Affiliation of Crystal Healing Organizations
c/o I.C.C.H
46 Lower Green Rd
Esher
Surrey KT10 8HD

The Reiki Association
Cornbrook Bridge House
Cornbrook, Clee Hill, Ludlow
Shropshire SY8 3Q

Holistic Association of Reflexologists
92 Sheering Rd
Old Harrow
Essex CM17 0JW

Association of Reflexologists
27 Old Gloucester St
London W1N 3XX
(for general information about reflexology)

The Register of Qualified Aromatherapists
PO Box 6941
London N8 9HF
(for a list of registered therapists)

The Aromatherapy Trades Council
PO Box 38
Romford
Essex RM1 2DNI
(for a list of essential oil suppliers)

Yoga Therapy Centre
Royal London Homoeopathic Hospital
60 Great Ormond St
London WC1N 3HR
(for information on yoga therapy and teacher training)

Yoga for Health Foundation
Ickwell Bury
Biggleswade
Bedfordshire SSG18 9EFl
(yoga centre offering courses)

INDEX

A

adrenalin 14, 15
adrenals 14, 16, 31, 37, 65
affirmation(s) 29, 138
    Crown 131; Heart 89; Root
    47; Sacral 61; Solar Plexus
    75; Third Eye 117; Throat
    103
agate 37, 44, 45, 93
aggressiveness 65
Air 31, 77, 78
Ajna 30, 105-17
allergies 33, 65
alligator 32, 51
altar(s) 24, 138
  Crown 124-5; Heart 82-3; Root
  41; Sacral 54-5; Solar Plexus
  68-9; Third Eye 110-11; Throat
  96-7
Alzheimer's 33, 121
amethyst 32, 107, 114, 121,
  128, 129
Anahata 30, 77-89
animals 32, 51, 65, 79, 93
antelope 32, 79
anti-depressants 128
anxiety 44
aquamarine 32, 93, 100, 129
Aquarius 31
archetype(s) 23, 32, 138
    Crown 121, 122-3; Heart 79,
    80-1; Root 37, 38-9; Sacral
    51, 52-3; Solar Plexus 65, 66-
    7; Third Eye 107, 108-9;
    Throat 93, 94-5
Aries 31
aromatherapy 132, 134
arrogance 92, 106
arthritis 25
asthma 25, 33, 93
astrology 135-7
    signs 31
aura 10, 12, 18-19, 138
auto-immune system 15
autonomic nervous system 14
aventurine quartz 79, 86
azurite 32, 79, 107, 114

B

back pain 33, 51
balancing chakras/energy 15,
    132, 134
Baptism 33, 37
behavioural patterns 23, 29
bergamot 32, 65, 79
betrayal 33, 79
bioelectromagnetic field 18, 19
Birth 16
bladder 31, 49, 51
    problems 33, 51
blockages 11, 72
    creative 33, 93, see also dys-
    functions
bloodstone 32, 37, 44
blue 30, 91, 92
body clock 16
bones 31, 37
brain 16, 17, 18
breathing problems 33, 79
Bridge pose 42-3
bull 32, 93
bullying 37

C

calcite 72, 73, 107, 114
calcium levels 15
calming mind and body 28, 100
Cancer 31, 33, 79
Capricorn 31
carbohydrates 33, 65
carnation 65
carnelian 32, 51, 58
cedarwood 32, 37
celestite 93, 100, 121, 129
central nervous system 17
cerebral cortex 31, 121
chakra system 8-11
    balancing 20-33, 132
chamomile 32, 93
charisma 106
Chart of Correspondences 30-3
chest 31, 79
chi 18, 132
chronic exhaustion/fatigue 33,
    65, 121
cinnamon 65
circulatory system 31, 49, 51, 79
citrine 32, 51, 58
clairaudience 100
cleansing crystals 27

clear quartz 32, 73, 121, 128
co-dependency 33, 79, 81
colour visualizations 112-13
colours 30, 32, 92, 106, 120
commitment 79
communication 15, 30, 91, 93,
    100, 119
Communicator 32, 93, 94-5
Communion 33, 51
compassion 33, 53, 77, 78, 80
Confession 33, 93
Confirmation 33, 65
confusion 33, 121
consciousness 10, 11, 100, 105
    higher 119, 135
contentedness 92
correspondences
    Crown 114, 121; Heart 78-9;
    Root 36-7; Sacral 50-1; Solar
    Plexus 64-5; Third Eye 106-7;
    Throat 92-3
Correspondences Chart 30-3
cosmic energy 31, 119, 120
courage 65
creativity 49, 51, 93, 100-1, 136
    blockages 33, 93
criticism 33, 65
Crown (7th) Chakra 16, 17,
    30-3, 114, 119-31, 137
crystal healing 26-7
crystals 32, 37, 51, 121, Crown
    128-9; cleansing 27; Heart
    79, 86-7; Root 44-5; Sacral
    58-9; Solar Plexus 65, 72-3;
    Third Eye 107, 114-15;
    Throat 93, 100-1; tuning 27

D

Daily Questions 28-9
    Crown 131; Heart 89; Root
    47; Sacral 61; Solar Plexus
    75; Third Eye 117; Throat
    103
decision-making 44
defence mechanisms 22
depression 33, 121
Descartes, René 16
detoxification 44
developmental ages 33, 37, 51,
    65, 79, 93
diabetes 15, 33, 65
diamond 32, 121, 128

digestive system 15, 31, 65, 66
    problems 33, 65, 66, 72
dis-ease 19
DNA 18
dogmatism 92, 106
dream/dreaming 87, 100
Drudge 32, 65, 66-7
dysfunctions 11, 20, 26, 138
    emotional/physical 15, 33,
    37, 51, 65, 79, 93, 107, 121

E, F
ears 31, 93
Earth 31, 35, 36
Earth Mother 32, 37, 38, 38-9,
    39
Edison, Thomas 108
effectiveness 65
Egocentric 32,121, 122-3
Einstein, Albert 108
elements 31, 63, 92, 105, 106,
    120
    air 77, 78; earth 35; fire 64;
    water 49, 50
elephant 32, 37, 93
emerald 79
emotions 22, 23
    balance 30, 51; blockages
    44; dysfunctions 33, 51, 65,
    79, 93, 107, 121; instability
    33, 51
endocrine system 12-13, 138
endurance 65
energy 12-19
    balancing 134; fields 10, 18;
    pathways 135
epilepsy 33, 121
essential oils 132, 134 see also
    oils
ether 31, 92
exercises
    Crown 126-7; Heart 84-5;
    meditation 27; physical 25;
    Root 42-3; Sacral 56-7; Solar
    Plexus 70-1; Third Eye 112-
    13; Throat 98-9
exhaustion 33, 73, 120
Extreme Unction 33, 121
eyes 31, 107
family identity 37
fantasism 50
fasting 33, 121

fatigue 25, 33
fears 33, 36, 53, 78, 79, 81
fire 31, 64
fire agate 44
Fitzgerald, Dr William 134
fluorite 32, 107
focusing 128
foods 33, 37, 51, 65, 79, 93
forgiveness 33, 77, 80
fragrances 32
frankincense 32, 121
free will 22, 23
frigidity 33, 50, 51
fruits 33, 93

G
garnet 37
gazelle 32, 79
Gemini 31
Genesis 17
genetic code 19
glands 12, 14, 31, 51, 79, 93,
    107, 121
glandular fever 94
glaucoma 33, 107
gold 30, 120
golden topaz 32, 51, 58, 129
gonads 16
gravity 35
green 30, 78
green calcite 79, 86
green jade 86
grounding 37, 42-3, 44, 138
group behaviour 38
Guru 32, 121, 122-3

H, I
habit forming 29
hallucinations 33, 107
happiness 81
harmony 30, 93, 100
headaches 33, 107
Headstand 126-7
healing energy 11, 26, 128
hearing 31, 91
    problems 93
heart 31, 79
    problems 25, 33, 79
Heart (4th) Chakra 15, 30-3, 77-
    89, 136
Heart Connection Exercise 84-5
hematite 32, 37, 44, 45

Herkimer diamond 121, 125,
    128
high blood pressure 25, 33, 79
Higher Self 17, 100, 128, 129,
    130, 135, 138
Hinduism 35, 49
hormones 12, 14, 15
human aura see aura
Hunt, Dr Valerie V. 18
hyacinth 32, 107
hypothalamus 16
imagination 108
impotence 33, 50, 51
incense 32, 37, 51, 65, 79, 93,
    107, 121
inconsistency 92
indigo 30, 106, 114
individuality 65
inner stillness 33, 37
inspiration 100
instability, emotional 33
intelligence, emotional 33
inter-connectedness 119
intuition/intuitiveness 16, 30,
    105, 106, 114, 136
irritable bowel syndrome 69, 73
isolation 33, 51

J, K
jade 79, 121
jasmine 32, 51
journal keeping 29
Jupiter 31, 106, 136
karma 20, 135
kidneys 44, 72
Kundalini 16-17, 35, 49, 119,
    128, 138

L, M
lapis lazuli 32, 93, 100, 107
lavender 32, 37, 121
learning difficulties 33, 107
left brain dominance 108, 115
Leo 31
lethargy, mental 33
Libra 31
life lessons 33
Light 31, 105, 106
Lingam 138
liquids 33, 51
liver 44
loneliness 79

lotus 35, 49, 64, 77, 78, 91, 92, 105, 106, 120
love 30, 77, 78, 79, 80, 85
Lover 32, 79, 80-1
lower back pain 33, 51
lungs 31, 79
lymphocytes 15
malachite 72, 73, 79, 129
mandalas 112-13, 138
manic depression 120
manipulation 50
Manipura 30, 63-75
Marriage 33, 79
Mars 31, 64, 136
Martyr 32, 51, 52-3
Masked Self 32, 93, 94-5
Mayan culture 86
meats 33, 37
meditation(s) 24, 27, 28, 50, 114, 128
    Crown 130-1; Heart 88-9; Root 46-7; Sacral 60-1; Solar Plexus 74-5; Third Eye 116-17; Throat 102-3
melancholia 33, 79
melatonin 16
melissa 32, 79
mental activity 100
    focusing 42-3; lethargy 33, 37
Mercury 31, 92, 136
meridians 135, 138
mind-body link 12
Moon 49
moonstone 58, 79
moss agate 44, 45
motherhood 16
motivations 33, 51
mouth 31, 93
Muladhara 30, 35-47
muscles 31, 65
musk 37
myrrh 32, 37, 93

N, O, P
neck 93, 94, 98
neckache 33, 93
negativity 44
Neptune 31, 106, 136
nervous system 14, 18
neural pathways 23, 29
neurological problems 33, 107

nightmares 33, 107
nose 93
objectivity 30, 93, 100
obsessions 33, 121
oils 32, 37, 51, 65, 79, 93, 107, 121
onyx 37
orange 30, 49, 50
Ordination 33, 107
osteoarthritis 33, 37
ovaries 14-15, 31, 51
over-activity 92
oversensitivity 33, 65
pancreas 14, 15, 31, 65, 72
parathyroid 15, 31, 93
partnerships 51
patchouli 32, 37
Pelvic Rock exercise 56-7
perfectionism 33, 93
Performer 32, 79, 80-1
personal expression 33
personal power 30, 65
physical
    dysfunctions 15, 33, 51, 65, 79, 93, 107, 121; exercises 25
physical health/fitness 37
physical needs 30, 37
pineal 14, 16, 31, 121
pink 30, 78
Pisces 31
pituitary 14, 16, 31, 107
planets 31, 64, 78, 92, 106, 120
Pluto 31, 50, 136
pollutants 33
possessiveness 79
prana 18
prostate 31, 51
proteins 33, 37
Psychic 32, 107, 108-9
psychic abilities 114
purple apartite 107
purple fluorite 114

Q, R
Qi 18
quartz 32, 37, 44, 58, 73, 79, 121, 129
ram 32, 65
Rationalist 32, 107, 108-9
red 30, 35, 36
Reflexology 134, 135
Reiki 134
rejection 53, 78

relationships 30, 79
reproductive organs 14-15, 49
rituals 24
Root (1st) Chakra 14, 17, 30-3, 35-47, 41, 134, 135
rose 32, 51, 65, 79
rose geranium 32, 107
rose quartz 37, 79, 86, 129
rosewood 32, 121
ruby 37

S
Sacral (2nd) Chakra 14-15, 30-3, 49-61, 136
    sacraments 33, 37, 51, 65, 79, 93, 107, 121
Sage 32, 121, 122-3
Sagittarius 31
Sahasrara 30, 119-31
sandalwood 32, 51
Sanskrit names and meanings 30
sapphire 93, 107
Saturn 31, 36, 135
schizophrenia 106
Scorpio 31
security 37, 44
self-centredness 37
self-confidence 33, 65
self-development 28-9
self-esteem 33, 37, 44, 64, 65, 66
self-expression 30, 93, 100
self-healing abilities 26
self-knowledge 93
self-pity 53, 78
self-respect 65
selflessness 33
self will 30, 65
senses 31, 37, 51, 65, 79, 93, 107
sensitivity 33, 121
setu bandhasara 42-3
sexual drives 33, 51
sexual organs 31, 49, 51
sexuality 14-15, 30, 51, 52
Shoulder Stand 98-9
shoulders 79
sight 31, 65
sixth sense 31, 107
skeletal structure 31, 37
skin 31, 121
skull 31, 107, 121

smell 31, 37
smoky quartz 37, 44, 45, 129
snowy quartz 121
sodalite 93, 100
Solar Plexus (3rd) Chakra 15,
    30-3, 63-75, 136
sore throat 33, 93, 94
sound 31, 93
Sovereign 32, 51, 52-3
spaciness 33, 37
speech 91
spinal cord 17
spiritual growth 23
Spiritual Warrior 32
spirituality 30
spleen 44, 72
stability 37
stamina 65
stimulants 100
stomach ulcers 15, 33, 65, 66,
    72
stress 25, 100
subtle body 12, 138
subtle energy system 8
Sun 31, 63, 64, 136
sunstone 32, 72
survival 30, 37
sushumna 10, 17, 112, 116, 138
Svadisthana 30, 49-61

T

taste 31, 51
Taurus 31
teeth 93
telepathic energy 31, 106
telepathy 136
tension 25
testes 14-15, 31, 51
therapies, integration 132-7
Third Eye (6th) Chakra 16, 17,
    25,30-3, 105-17, 136
thought 31, 119, 120
    as energy 12; patterns 29
throat 31, 93
Throat (5th) Chakra 15, 30-3,
    91-103, 136
thymus 14, 15, 31, 79
thyroid 14, 15, 16, 31, 93
    problems 33, 93, 94
thyroxine 15
tiger's eye 32, 37, 44, 45
tinnitus 33, 93
topaz see golden topaz
touch 31, 79
tourmaline see watermelon;
    white
tribal concept 36, 37, 38
tuning crystals 27
turquoise 32, 93, 100

U, V, W, Y, Z

unhappiness 52
Universal Life Force 11, 17, 18,
    20, 26, 132, 134, 138
Uranus 31, 120, 137
Vedas 11, 25
vegetables 33, 79
Venus 31, 78, 136
vetivert 32, 65
vibrational energy/healing 10,
    12, 26
Victim 32, 37, 38, 38-9, 39
violet 30, 32, 107, 120
Virgo 31
Vishuddha 30, 99-103
vision problems 33, 107
visualizations 28, 50, 70-1, 112-
    13
Warrior 65, 66-7
Water 31, 49, 50
watermelon tourmaline 32, 79,
    86
well-being 20, 25, 26
white 30, 120
white jade 121
white tourmaline 121
wisdom 30
womb 31, 51
yellow 30, 63, 64
yellow citrine 32, 72, 73
yin and yang 49, 138
ylang ylang 32, 65
yoga poses 25, 42-3, 98-9, 126-7
zodiacal signs 135
Zone Therapy 134

Author's Acknowledgements

I believe each of our relationships has something
to teach us about the chakras. These are the people to whom I am indebted for helping me to heal
and balance mine, and in doing so contributed to
the writing of this book:

Martine Delamere; Maggie Sapiets; Bonnie and
John McGrath; Paul Kitson; Caroline Faulkener;
Jean Taylor; Teresa Hale; Jo Godfrey Wood. And
certainly not least my children, Graeme and
Caroline, for showing me the meaning of uncon-
ditional love and keeping me grounded.

Publisher's Acknowledgements

Gaia Books would like to thank the following indi-
viduals for their contribution to this book: Sam
Dightam, Sarah Harris, Missak Takoushian, Sandi
Takoushian, Meriam Soopee (models), Mary
Warren (indexing and proofreading), Mark
Preston, Matt Moate, and all those who lent
props.

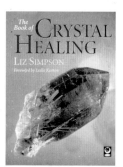
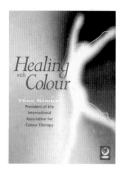
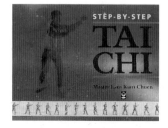
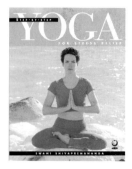
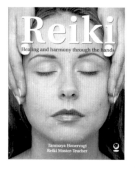